ADVANCES IN

Family Practice Nursing

Editor-in-Chief
Linda J. Keilman, DNP, MSN,
GNP-BC, FAANP

Associate Editors
Melodee Harris, PhD, RN, FAAN

Sharon L. Holley, DNP, CNM,
FACNM

Imelda Reyes, DNP, MPH, APRN,
CPNP-PC, FNP-BC, FAANP

PHILADELPHIA   LONDON   TORONTO   MONTREAL   SYDNEY   TOKYO

Editor: Kerry Holland
Developmental Editor: Hannah Almira Lopez

Editorial Office:
Elsevier
1600 John F. Kennedy Blvd,
Suite 1800
Philadelphia, PA 19103-2899

International Standard Serial Number: 2589-420X
International Standard Book Number: 978-0-323-98677-9

Editor-in-Chief

LINDA J. KEILMAN, DNP, MSN, GNP-BC, FAANP, Associate Professor, Gerontology Population Content Expert, Michigan State University, College of Nursing, East Lansing, Michigan

Associate Editors

MELODEE HARRIS, PHD, RN, FAAN, Co-Director, National Hartford Center of Gerontological Nursing Excellence, Reston, Virginia; Assistant Professor, College of Nursing, University of Arkansas for Medical Sciences, Little Rock, Arkansas

SHARON L. HOLLEY, DNP, CNM, FACNM, Director, Nurse-Midwifery Pathway, University of Alabama at Birmingham, Birmingham, Alabama

IMELDA REYES, DNP, MPH, APRN, CPNP-PC, FNP-BC, FAANP, Associate Clinical Professor, Pediatric Primary Care NP Program Director, Emory University, Nell Hodgson Woodruff School of Nursing, Atlanta, Georgia

CONTRIBUTORS

BETH A. AMMERMAN, DNP, FNP-BC, Clinical Assistant Professor, Department of Health Behavior and Biological Sciences, University of Michigan School of Nursing, Ann Arbor, Michigan

TAMATHA ARMS, PhD, DNP, PMHNP-BC, NP-C, University of North Carolina Wilmington, Associate Professor, CHHS School of Nursing, Wilmington, North Carolina

MAEGHAN E. ARNOLD, DNP, APRN, AGACNP-BC, Clinical Assistant Professor, College of Nursing University of Arkansas for Medical Sciences, Palliative and Supportive Medicine Nurse Practitioner, Baptist Health Medical Center, Little Rock, Arkansas

NICOLE LYNNE AUDRITSH, DNP, CNM, Wayne State University, Detroit, Michigan

SHARON BRONNER, DNP, GNP-BC, ACHPN, Clinical Educator, Centers Health Care, New York, New York

PAMELA Z. CACCHIONE, PhD, CRNP, BC, FSGA, University of Pennsylvania, School of Nursing, Philadelphia, Pennsylvania

REBECCA CLARK, DNP, RN, CNE, MEDSURG-BC, Assistant Professor, Texas Tech University Health Sciences Center, Lubbock, Texas

MICHELE DAVIDE, MS, APN, FNP-BC, Family Nurse Practitioner, Advocare, West Morris Pediatrics, Succasunna, New Jersey

LAURA C. FORD, PhD, RN, CNP, Certifications in Women's Health, Menopause Clinician, Sexual Therapy, Adjunct Faculty, Western Michigan University, Kalamazoo, Michigan

KATHARINE GREEN, PhD, CNM, FACNM, Director, Accelerated 2nd Bachelor's Program, College of Nursing, University of Massachusetts Amherst, Amherst, Massachusetts

MELODEE HARRIS, PhD, RN, FAAN, Associate Professor, College of Nursing, University of Arkansas for Medical Sciences, Little Rock, Arkansas

ELIZABETH HUTSON, PhD, APRN-CNP, PMHNP-BC, Associate Professor, Texas Tech University Health Sciences Center, School of Nursing, Lubbock, Texas

HEATHER M. JONES, DNP, AGPCNP-C, Clinical Assistant Professor, Department of Health Behavior and Biological Sciences, University of Michigan School of Nursing, Ann Arbor, Michigan

LINDA J. KEILMAN, DNP, MSN, GNP-BC, FAANP, Associate Professor, Gerontology Population Content Expert, Michigan State University, College of Nursing, East Lansing, Michigan

LAURIE KENNEDY-MALONE, PhD, GNP-BC, FAANP, FGSA, UNCG School of Nursing, Greensboro, North Carolina

CHRISTIAN KETEL, DNP, RN, Vanderbilt University School of Nursing, Murfreesboro, Tennessee

ELIZABETH K. KUZMA, DNP, FNP-BC, Clinical Assistant Professor, Department of Health Behavior and Biological Sciences, University of Michigan School of Nursing, Ann Arbor, Michigan

PAMELA J. LaBORDE, DNP, APRN, CCNS, TTS, University of Arkansas for Medical Sciences, Clinical Assistant Professor, College of Nursing, Little Rock, Arkansas

AMY M. LEWITZ, MS, APRN, PMHCNS, Lincolnwood, Illinois

MAUD LOW, PhD, RNC, CLNC, Clinical Assistant Professor, College of Nursing, University of Massachusetts Amherst, Amherst, Massachusetts

RHONDA WELLS LUCAS, MSN, AGPCNP-BC, GS-C, Optum HouseCalls, Elkridge, Maryland

KAREN DEVEREAUX MELILLO, PhD, A-GNP-C, FAANP, FGSA, Solomont School of Nursing, Zuckerberg College of Health Sciences, University of Massachusetts Lowell, Lowell, Massachusetts

LISA MILITELLO, PhD, MPH, RN, CPNP, Assistant Professor, The Ohio State University, College of Nursing, Ohio

DONNA MARSHALL MOYER, PhD, RN, PCNS-BC, Assistant Professor, Michigan State University, College of Nursing, East Lansing, Michigan

CECILIA A. NWOGU, DNP, GNP-BC, PMHNP, Adult Health Consultant of Atlanta Inc, Conyers, Georgia

GEORGE BYRON PERAZA-SMITH, DNP, GNP-BC, AGPCNP-C, CNE, APRN-BC, GS-C, FAANP, Nursing Department Chair, DNP and APRN Online Programs, South University, Savannah, Georgia

MARY LAUREN PFIEFFER, DNP, FNP-BC, Assistant Professor, Vanderbilt University School of Nursing, Nashville, Tennessee

JENNIFER C. RISKE, BSN, RN, OCN, Department of Health Behavior and Biological Sciences, University of Michigan School of Nursing, Ann Arbor, Michigan

KATIE SCARLETT, CCLS, Child Life Educator, Children's Healthcare of Atlanta, Atlanta, Georgia

ANN SHEEHAN, DNP, CPNP, FAANP, Interim Director for Faculty Practice and Assistant Professor Health Professions, Michigan State University, College of Nursing, East Lansing, Michigan

JENNA SMITH, LCSW, MSSW, Vanderbilt University Medical Center, Goodlettsville, Tennessee

WILLIS SMITH, MSN, PMHNP-BC, LPC, Vanderbilt University Medical Center, Nashville, Tennessee

JANICE TAYLOR, DNP, AGPCNP-BC, UAMS College of Nursing, Little Rock, Arkansas

MEGHAN TRACEWSKI, MSN, RN, CPNP, ACHPN, Palliative Care Nurse Practitioner, Pediatric Advanced Care Team, Children's Healthcare of Atlanta

CANDICE VADEN, MSN, WHNP-BC, AGPCNP-BC, Vanderbilt University School of Nursing, Franklin, Tennessee

VALLON WILLIAMS, DNP, APRN, AGNP-C, Clinical Research Nurse Practitioner, University of Arkansas for Medical Sciences, Translational Research Institute, Research Department

Linda J. Keilman, Melodee Harris, Sharon L. Holley, and
Imelda Reyes

ADULT/GERIATRIC

Rebecca Clark

Older adults experience many challenges and can benefit from a
whole health approach to care that includes mental healthcare.
Mental health screening tools for depression and anxiety
specific to the older adult population can be incorporated into
practice with planning. Three validated tools for depression in
the geriatric population discussed are the Geriatric Depression
Scale, the Patient Health Questionnaire, and the Cornell Scale
for Depression in Dementia. The Geriatric Anxiety Inventory
is a screening tool for anxiety for the later-life older adult
population. Screening for depression and anxiety can improve
the quality of life.

The Surprising Effects of Social Isolation and Loneliness on Physical Health in Older Adults

Pamela J. LaBorde and Vallon Williams

This article highlights the physical impact of social isolation and loneliness in older adults and discusses 3 central physical systems affected by these conditions. In addition, information is provided regarding social isolation and loneliness related to components of assessment, appropriate preventive interventions, the impact on health care utilization, and the role of the advanced practice nurse in addressing social isolation and loneliness in the elderly population.

The Mental Health and Well Being of Older Adults in Hospice and Palliative Care

Maeghan E. Arnold

Hospice and palliative care are interdisciplinary services focused on holistic treatment of patients with advanced, life-limiting illnesses. In addition to physiologic manifestations of chronic illnesses, patients are at higher risk for depression, anxiety, and spiritual distress. These issues negatively influence quality of life and well-being. Health care providers' frequent use of assessment tools (ie, Functional Assessment Staging Tool, Palliative Performance Scale, Eastern Cooperative Oncology Group Performance Status, and New York Heart Association Functional Classification) may guide earlier referral to palliative care or hospice services. Patients who receive palliative care have demonstrated improved depression, anxiety, and quality of life.

Culturally Informed Mental Health Care of Marginalized Older Adults   37

Tamatha Arms, Linda J. Keilman, and
George Byron Peraza-Smith

Culturally informed care should be the foundation of every professional encounter with patients, whether that culture is different from the health care providers (HCP) or not. Taking the time to understand how different cultures view health, and in particular mental health, can only help stabilize and strengthen the patient–provider relationship. A strong therapeutic relationship is particularly important when interacting with marginalized older adults diagnosed with a mental health condition. In this article, marginalization includes older adults who are members of an ethnic minority population, immigrants to the United States, military veterans, live with an intellectual/developmental disorder (I/DD), or identify as LGBTQ + meaning lesbian/gay/bisexual/transgender/queer (or sometimes questioning); the plus represents other gender identities and sexual orientations. The world population is changing and expanding. Without accurate cultural understanding and knowledge, HCPs cannot accurately diagnose or treat patients at the highest standard of care.

The Medicare Wellness Visit: A Time to Address Mental Health and Well-Being   55

Rhonda Wells Lucas, Janice Taylor, and
Laurie Kennedy-Malone

The Medicare Annual Wellness Visit (AWV) provides an opportunity each year for health care providers of older adults and disabled persons to spend time comprehensively reviewing risk factors and indicators of common problems faced by this population. Multiple components of the AWV pertain to a patient's mental health and well-being. By providing a written personalized plan that not only includes updates for immunizations and preventative screenings but addresses sensitive issues such as memory, depression, life satisfaction, stress, anger, loneliness, social isolation, pain, and fatigue, nurse practitioners can assist the person in being proactive in working toward better health outcomes.

Basic Considerations for Understanding and Treating Delirium Psychosis in Older Adults

Cecilia A. Nwogu, Linda J. Keilman, George Byron Peraza-Smith, Pamela Z. Cacchione, Sharon Bronner, Karen Devereaux Melillo, Amy M. Lewitz, Tamatha Arms, and Melodee Harris

Delirium psychosis is common in older adults. Although the Diagnostic and Statistical Manual (DSM) provides criteria for delirium, there are no specific criteria for older adults. Older adults with delirium psychosis present atypically. If the underlying cause is not diagnosed and treated, delirium can result in permanent cognitive deficits. Prevention of delirium is paramount. First-line treatment of delirium includes nonpharmacological interventions. Atypical presentations include delirium superimposed on dementia, psychosis associated with Charles Bonnet Syndrome, and terminal psychosis at the end of life.

WOMEN'S HEALTH

Integrating Behavioral Health into Primary Care for Women   79

Jenna Smith, Candice Vaden, Willis Smith, and Christian Ketel

Mental illness is prevalent across the United States and is often brought to health care providers' attention in regular and follow-ups visits. Barriers to mental health care include identification of mental health needs, provider comfort, access or availability to care, delays in receiving counseling services, and patients lost in transition to specialty mental health services. Behavioral health integration involves incorporating these services directly into the health care setting. The ability for providers to collaborate with the behavioral health team allows for the creation of cohesive treatment plans and retention of patients who may otherwise be lost to follow-up.

The Well-Woman Visit: Adolescence Through End-of-Life   91

Beth A. Ammerman, Heather M. Jones, Jennifer C. Riske, and Elizabeth K. Kuzma

This article outlines the key components of the well-woman visit for all women, beginning with a comprehensive health history, a complete head to toe physical examination, routine screening recommendations, immunizations, as well as health counseling and anticipatory guidance. It further outlines the unique components to each of these elements for 3 distinct age groups: adolescents aged 12 through 21 years, women older than 21 through 64 years, and women 65 years and older. This article is meant to be used as a tool for practicing primary care nurse practitioners to guide their care of the well-woman.

Recurrent Vulvovaginal Candidiasis: Implications for Practice

Mary Lauren Pfieffer

Vaginal symptoms are a frequent chief complaint seen in women. These symptoms are related to vulvovaginal candidiasis (VVC) 40% of the time. Recurrent and chronic vulvovaginal candidiasis are also seen in patients with unremitting, chronic symptoms. Misdiagnosis and underdiagnosis of VVC occurs often. It is important women's health care providers are up to date on guidelines for assessing, diagnosing, and treating VVC.

Genitourinary Syndrome of Menopause: Assessment and Management Options 131
Laura C. Ford

Genitourinary syndrome ofmenopause (GSM) is a hypoestrogenic condition inclusive of complaints of genital discomfort, sexual dysfunction, and urinary signs and symptoms. GSM differs from vulvovaginal atrophy because it is inclusive of urinary complaints of incontinence, altered bladder capacity, and change in the urinary and vaginal microbiome. This article educates the primary care clinician providing women's health care to enhance diagnosis and treatment of GSM because "it is essential to recognize and treat this syndrome in order to restore the vaginal and vulvar epithelium and ultimately improve quality of life" for the postmenopausal women entrusted to our care.

Postpartum Depression: Updates in Evaluation and Care 145
Katharine Green and Maud Low

Depression and anxiety, both risk factors for peripartum depression including postpartum depression, have increased during the COVID-19 pandemic. With the increased risks of postpartum depression to birthing parents, their newborns, and their families, advanced practice nurses need to be aware of the incidence, screening tools, and treatments for this disorder. Recommendations include the screening of all pregnant and postpartum patients including during pediatric visits, encouraging support postpartum, and teaching patients families to recognize the symptoms of postpartum depression and report them to their care providers.

Measuring the Impact of Health Literacy on Perinatal Depression

Nicole Lynne Audritsh

Depression is the third leading cause of disease burden in the world for women, and individuals with low health literacy are 2 times more likely to experience depression symptoms than individuals with adequate health literacy skills. Major or minor depression during pregnancy, or during the postpartum period of the first 12 months following delivery, is diagnosed as perinatal depression. Health literacy is the degree to which an individual can obtain, process, and understand the basic health information and services they need to make informed and appropriate health-related decisions.

PEDIATRICS

The Good, the Bad, and the Potential: Best Practices for Navigating Technology Use Among Pediatric Populations

Lisa Militello and Elizabeth Hutson

An honest dialogue regarding how children and teens continue to use various technologies is critical to pediatric primary care and health supervision. Technology use among children and teens exceeds current guidelines. The authors highlight opportunities for health care providers to reconcile expert recommendations with real-world technology use. Providers are encouraged to assess technology use in families, identify both positive and at-risk behaviors, and guide positive technology adoption among children, teens, and families.

Treating Adolescent Anxiety and Depression in Primary Care Considering Pandemic Mental Health Fallout

Michele Davide

Child health experts have been studying pediatric mental illness for decades. Research quantifying high rates of pediatric mental illness along with a shortage of specialty providers demonstrated a need for change. Pediatric advocacy organizations encouraged pediatric primary care providers to offer a basic level of treatment for mild to moderate mental health symptoms in the primary care setting to help offset the pediatric mental health provider shortage and allow specialists to focus on patients with more severe symptoms. Fallout from the COVID-19 pandemic increased rates of pediatric mental illness, especially adolescent depression and anxiety. The time has come for pediatric primary care providers to embrace mental wellness in their practices, implement research-based interventions, break down barriers to treatment, and do their part to fight the National Children's Mental Health Emergency ignited by the COVID-19 pandemic.

Grief in Children 203

Meghan Tracewski and Katie Scarlett

The primary care provider is an important resource to a family impacted by death. Children can be left out of the grieving process owing to misperceptions around their ability to understand and navigate their complex emotions. This article reviews theories of grief and the process of acclimating to life without the deceased as it pertains to a child's developmental conceptualization and comprehension of death. This article offers a framework for assessing family coping to best support the grieving child and tools to improve provider comfort in navigating difficult discussions with the pediatric patient.

Mind-Body Therapies for Children with Functional Abdominal Pain   **217**

Donna Marshall Moyer and Ann Sheehan

Functional abdominal pain (FAP) is a common condition of children and adolescents and is associated with several negative physical and psychological health outcomes. Because the diagnosis of FAP is based on symptomatology and no structural or physiologic cause is identified, it can be difficult to manage. There is emerging and growing evidence that supports the role of mind-body therapies in a successful plan of care. In this article, the authors provide an overview of some promising mind-body therapies and make recommendations for their use in care of pediatric patients with functional abdominal pain.

PREFACE

Lessons Learned as the Global Pandemic Lingers

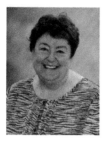 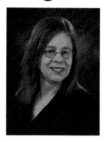 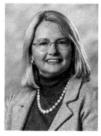 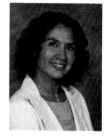

Linda J. Keilman, DNP, MSN, GNP-BC, FAANP

Melodee Harris, PhD, RN, FAAN

Sharon L. Holley, DNP, CNM, FACNM

Imelda Reyes, DNP, MPH, APRN, CPNP-PC, FNP-BC, FAANP

Editors

I t was March 11, 2020 when the World Health Organization declared a global pandemic related to the worldwide spread of the novel coronavirus COVID-19.[1] It is now 2022, and the world continues to reel from the devastation the pandemic has caused in so many ways. At the writing of this preface, the world is experiencing a variant of concern: Omicron B.1.1.529, first identified in South Africa.[2] Viruses are constantly changing and mutating, resulting in new variants of the original. Omicron is to date the fastest spreading new COVID-19 variant across the United States; people are susceptible to contracting the virus even when fully vaccinated. As reported by CBS News on January 4, 2022, the Omicron variant was responsible for approximately 95.4% of new COVID-19 cases in the first week of the new year.[3] Many people in the United States were trying to get tested for the variant: schedules did not match up with offered times; lines were long; people were desperate. A lesson learned from the pandemic has been how could citizens receive quicker, efficient testing for the virus to decrease stress and fear and to early quarantine if positive? Free at-home COVID-19 tests are now available in the United States at https://www.covidtests.gov/.[4] There is a simple fill-in application process online, and four kits arrive in the mailbox via the US Postal Service. This

https://doi.org/10.1016/j.yfpn.2022.01.002
2589-420X/22/© 2022 Published by Elsevier Inc.

is a terrific advancement in detection and management of the disease; a good lesson to come out of the pandemic!

Fortunately, there have been other lessons learned from the devastation! The health inequities and disparities experienced by older adults, minorities, marginalized/vulnerable individuals, those with low socioeconomic status, and those with mental health disorders came to the forefront in publicly exposing the gaps and flaws in the US health care system. According to the National Alliance on Mental Illness,[5] one in five adults in the United States experience mental illness. In addition, approximately 70% of youth in the juvenile justice system have a mental health diagnosis, and 18.8% of high school students have thought seriously about suicide.[5]

Health care professionals are being challenged to ignite the flame of transformation now and begin implementing visionary and innovative changes for the future. Change begins with each human being: self-reflection, mindfulness, and moving away from tunnel vision to a better understanding of self and others. One way to move forward as individuals is to learn more about how culture impacts every human being in different ways. It is through seeking new knowledge, doing honest self-evaluation, and envisioning a better health care system that change can begin.

Another way to learn more lessons is to read about what is currently occurring in health care being provided by Advanced Practice Registered Nurses (APRN) across the country. In this year's edition of *Advances in Family Practice Nursing*, you will find information that covers care across the lifespan, from pediatrics through gerontology, from birth to death. A wide range of subjects are covered by the authors, such as depression, anxiety, social isolation, loneliness, mental health and well-being until the end of life, culturally informed care, wellness visits, delirium psychosis, and health literacy; there are also articles covering vulvovaginal candidiasis; menopause in women; and bullying, sleep, fatigue, grief, and abdominal pain in children. Many of the articles reflect on the presence of COVID-19 and how health care has incorporated the pandemic into current APRN practice clinical review.

The editors and authors hope these articles will spark awareness of the depth and breadth of the novel coronavirus and its variants and the lingering impact on daily life, including mental health. Understanding the current health care climate and culture is important for all APRN to understand as it impacts the lives of human beings. The United States cannot go back to prepandemic health care; too much has been learned to try and fix an archaic, broken system. Innovation is the key; learning and moving toward a brighter future of health for all is the path that APRN should take as we move forward in the year 2022.

Linda J. Keilman, DNP, MSN, GNP-BC, FAANP
Gerontology Population Content Expert
Michigan State University, College of Nursing
1355 Bogue Street, A126

Life Sciences Building
East Lansing, MI 48824-1317, USA

E-mail address: keilman@msu.edu

Melodee Harris, PhD, RN, FAAN
University of Arkansas for Medical Sciences
College of Nursing
4301 West Markham Street, Slot #529
Little Rock, AR 72205, USA

E-mail address: HarrisMelodee@uams.edu

Sharon L. Holley, DNP, CNM, FACNM
Nurse-Midwifery Pathway
University of Alabama at Birmingham
1701 University Boulevard
Birmingham, AL 35294, USA

E-mail address: sharonholley@uab.edu

Imelda Reyes, DNP, MPH, APRN, CPNP-PC, FNP-BC, FAANP
Pediatric Primary Care
Emory University
Nell Hodgson Woodruff School of Nursing
1520 Clifton Road, Suite 432
Atlanta, GA 30322, USA

E-mail address: imelda.reyes@emory.edu

REFERENCES

1 Cucinotta D, Vanelli M. WHO declares COVID-19 a pandemic. Acta Biomed 2020;91(1):157–60.
2 Centers for Disease Control and Prevention. What you need to know about variants. 2021. Available at: https://www.cdc.gov/coronavirus/2019-ncov/variants/about-variants.html?CDC_AA_refVal=https%3A%2F%2Fwww.cdc.gov%2Fcoronavirus%2F2019-ncov%2Fvariants%2Fvariant.html#print. Accessed January 22, 2022.
3 Tin A. Omicron now 95% of new COVID-19 infection in U.S., CDC estimates. CBS News. 2022. Available at: https://www.covidtests.gov/. Accessed January 22, 2022.
4 United States Government. Get free at-home COVID-19 tests. Available at: https://www.covidtests.gov/. Accessed January 22, 2022.
5 National Alliance on Mental Illness. Mental health by the numbers. 2021. Available at: https://www.nami.org/mhstats. Accessed January 22, 2022.

Adult/Geriatric

Older Adults and Late-Life Depression and Anxiety Screening

Choices in Care for Optimal Outcomes of Mental Health

Rebecca Clark, DNP, RN, CNE, MEDSURG-BC*

Texas Tech University Health Sciences Center, 3601 4th street, STOP 6264, Lubbock, TX 79430-6264, USA

Keywords
- Mental health • Older adults • Later-life older adults • Geriatrics • Screening tools
- Long-term care • Geriatric depression scale

Key points

- For older adults, failure to address late-life depression and anxiety results in decreased quality of life.
- Depression and anxiety screening tools are beneficial in determining the care an older adult may need.
- Having a clear workflow for screening tool follow-up will reduce reluctance and increase the incorporation of screening tools into practice.
- Screening tools should be specific to the setting practice, population, and diagnoses of the older adult.

INTRODUCTION

Despite older adults' experiences with multiple losses and changes, mental health is frequently not addressed. Mental health assessment can be challenging in primary care practice for older adults with multiple chronic conditions [1]. Challenges include access to care from provider availability to transportation and cost, social determinants of health, stigma, and lack of understanding of mental health in older adults. Mental health diagnoses such as depression,

*4409 88th Street, Lubbock, TX 79424. *E-mail address:* rebecca.clark@ttuhsc.edu

https://doi.org/10.1016/j.yfpn.2021.12.014
2589-420X/22/© 2022 Elsevier Inc. All rights reserved.

anxiety, and dementia are not a planned part of aging. However, mental health has become a focus in the whole health model of care, with the goal of mental health care being provided from initial contact and interwoven throughout the lifespan. The American Psychiatric Nurses Association's (APNA) position statement supports mental health as the starting point to whole health, health promotion, and early identification, along with access to and proper treatment. APNA also highlights screening as an essential component of adequate mental health care [2]. Failure to address mental health can lead to a decreased quality of life, increased suffering, and physical and social decline [3].

This chapter focuses on screening tools for late-life depression and anxiety in older adults supported by the influx in depression and anxiety in this population. Twenty percent of older adults experience a mental health disorder [3]. Of those meeting criteria for a mental health diagnosis, less than 40% receive treatment. Suicidal ideation is 48 times higher in older adults with depression screenings that indicate moderately severe depression [4]. These statistics support and resonate the importance of screening tools.

According to the Centers for Disease Control and Prevention (CDC), 8% of older adults report acute depression and 16% chronic depression in individuals older than 50 years [5]. Demographics influence incidence. Depression ranges vary by location for patients older than 65 years. Patients residing in the community have the lowest rate at 1% to 5%, add in-home health care services, and the rate increases to greater than 13%. The highest incidence occurs in long-term and assisted care facilities at 25% [5,6]. Anxiety in older adults occurs at a 10% to 20% incidences. Most of the later-life anxiety is mild, and 2% of older adult–diagnosed anxiety is severe [5].

The Diagnostic and Statistical Manual of Mental Disorders-5 (DSM-5) has 8 criteria for depression. An individual must experience at least 5 symptoms during 2 continuous weeks. Loss of pleasure or interest or deflated mood must be one of the required criteria. See Box 1 for criteria for depression. The symptoms must substantially affect the individual regarding their relationships, ability to function, and activities of daily living and must not be attributed to a substance abuse problem or other medical diagnoses [7]. Late-life criteria are absent, and more research specific to this age group is needed. Depression and anxiety can present together [8]. Symptomology can be masked by other disease processes such as dementia and be overlooked [9].

Mental health disorders are a public health crisis, and screening is underutilized [3]. By 2030, an estimated 15 million adults older than 65 years will have a mental illness, a mental health disorder, or a substance abuse issue [10]. In Quick Facts of the National Coalition on Mental Health and Aging, completed suicide rates of white men 85 years and older occur 4 times society's rate. Overall, the suicide rate is nearly 6 times higher in later-life older adults in the United States, accounting for one of the highest incidences of suicide, comprising 20% of total suicides [4,10]. Mental health also affects health care costs. Health care expenditures are increased on average 50% more in individuals 65 years and older with a mental health diagnosis [11].

Box 1: Diagnostic and Statistical Manual of Mental Disorders criteria for depression

1. A depressed mood for most of the day occurring almost every day
2. Disinterest or no pleasure from daily activities for most of the day, nearly every day
3. Weight loss or weight gain is significant, and appetite is markedly increased or decreased almost daily
4. Thought processes and reaction time decrease; observable by the provider
5. Daily or almost daily fatigue or loss of energy
6. Guilty feelings or feeling worthless nearly every day
7. Being indecisive and having a decreased capacity for thinking or concentrating
8. Thoughts of death and suicide ideation are recurrent. Suicide has been attempted in the past, has a plan for suicide

°Older adults are not explicitly addressed in the criteria.

Data from Truschel, Jessica. Depression definition and DSM-5 diagnostic criteria. In Pyscom. 2020. https://www.psycom.net/depression-definition-dsm-5-diagnostic-criteria/. Accessed on August on August 31, 2021.

The older adult population receives services in various settings, including outpatient facilities such as home health and community care, inpatient acute care settings, long-term care facilities, and primary care settings. Therefore, it is essential to explore and address screening tools appropriate for these various settings. Providers can examine screening tools and develop an algorithm for efficient screening and referrals specific to their practice area. For example, through a systematic review, 4 Geriatric Depression Scales (GDS) were beneficial for detecting depression in older adults. However, the more concise versions of the GDS, such as GDS 15 and 10, had higher sensitivity and specificity [12].

OLDER ADULT SCREENING TOOLS

In older adults, mental and physical health are interwoven. The more physical ailments a person has, the more likely they also have a mental illness and vice versa in this age group [5]. Because this patient population seeks care, an appropriate screening tool needs to be in place to assess their mental health. Tools are available specific to screening older adults with late-life depression or anxiety in various settings. Table 1 provides multiple tools with free apps or Web sites for easy incorporation into practice.

BENEFITS, BARRIERS, AND GAPS TO SCREENING

Incorporating screening into practice has positive outcomes, including improving quality of life and decreasing overall health care expenses [2]. The combined impact of multiple medical diagnoses and worsening of mental health diagnoses drops when screening with validated tools and systematic plans are in place for

Table 1
Helpful Web sites to access content

Tool Name	Brief Description	Web Site	What You'll Find	Additional Info
GDS-15	Geriatric Depression Scale	https://web.stanford.edu/~yesavage/GDS.html	Page contains free phone apps and desktop webpage to incorporate into your practice	Available on this page in many languages (not all languages validated)
US Preventive Task Force (USPSTF) Screening Tool	Assists in choosing screening tools	https://www.uspreventiveservicestaskforce.org/apps/	Accessed as an app for your phone or webpage, it contains a rationale, general and clinical info, and tools	All USPSTF screening tools populate when you add specific demographic information about your patient
Pfizer Patient Health Questionnaire	PHQ (various forms) and GAD	https://www.phqscreeners.com/select-screener	Free to use and reproduce for practice, available in multiple languages	Includes various PHQ-Brief, 4, 8, 9, 15, SADS, and GAD-7 with an instruction manual
Geriatric Anxiety Inventory (GAI)	Explanation on how to access screening tool	http://gai.net.au/	Cost for providers, free for academia, both require permission	Web site includes way to obtain license (permission) history and use

follow-up [5]. The Center for Medicare & Medicaid Services (CMS), require yearly metrics of depression readmission rates that affect reimbursement. CMS couples readmission rates with a Patient Health Questionnaire-9 score greater than 9 [13].

The United States Preventive Services Task Force (USPSTF) recommends screening for all adults regardless of chief complaint or medical history. However, some risk factors that warrant a heightened need for screening include a past diagnosis of depression, loneliness, chronic disease processes affecting the quality of life, disability, sleep issues, and complicated grief [1,5,14].

Provider time constraints are a barrier to the utilization of screening tools in practice. Most screening tools can be self-administered depending on the client's ability and having a caregiver present if the client cannot complete the screening tool. The screening tool is often completed during the time the patient waits to see their provider. Follow-up can also hinder the administration of a screening tool. Another barrier is knowing what steps or algorithms to follow if a patient has a positive result from their screening tool. Stigma is also a barrier, and the significance of mental health stigma can contribute to a client not being forthcoming or declining completion or follow-up of a positive screening tool [3].

DEPRESSION SCREENING TOOLS

Mr J has middle-stage Alzheimer disease coupled with vision and hearing impairment. His caregiver reports that he has been having angry outbursts and extreme frustration, followed by periods where he withdraws from his family and becomes sullen and temperamental. He confuses words, and during your interview, it is not easy to ascertain his take on what he is experiencing. Physically, his assessment is unremarkable, but his mental health raises red flags. The provider recognized criteria for depression from the DSM-5 and decides screening for depression is warranted. See Box 1 for the DSM-5 criteria for depression list. Options discussed in detail are the Geriatric Depression Scale, Patient Health Questionnaire, and the Cornell Scale for Depression. Each is discussed in the following section.

The GDS is available in several versions: GDS-30, also known as the GDS-Long (GDS-L), and the GDS-15, also known as the GDS-Short (GDS-S). See Fig. 1 for the GDS-Short screening tool and scoring instructions. These are differentiated by the number of screening questions. The original is the 30-item form, GDS-L. The most used and preferred is the 15-item form, GDS-S. The GDS can be self-administered or read to individuals. It has an average administration time of 5 to 10 minutes. Evidence supports its effectiveness for patients with aphasia using an answer board and patients with dementia due to its brevity. It has been validated in all settings for older adults [15].

The Patient Health Questionnaire (PHQ) is administered as a self-assessment. Validity and reliability, and internal consistency, are supported with evidence-based research. The PHQ is most commonly administered in its 2- or 9-question format; if the results are positive in the 2-question form, the best practice is to follow-up with the 9-question design [16]. The PHQ is also available and validated in many languages; it can be read to older adult clients when warranted.

Geriatric Depression Scale (GDS)
Scoring Instructions

Instructions: Score 1 point for each bolded answer. A score of 5 or more suggests depression.

1.	Are you basically satisfied with your life?	yes	**no**
2.	Have you dropped many of your activities and interests?	**yes**	no
3.	Do you feel that your life is empty?	**yes**	no
4.	Do you often get bored?	**yes**	no
5.	Are you in good spirits most of the time?	yes	**no**
6.	Are you afraid that something bad is going to happen to you?	**yes**	no
7.	Do you feel happy most of the time?	yes	**no**
8.	Do you often feel helpless?	**yes**	no
9.	Do you prefer to stay at home, rather than going out and doing things?	**yes**	no
10.	Do you feel that you have more problems with memory than most?	**yes**	no
11.	Do you think it is wonderful to be alive now?	yes	**no**
12.	Do you feel worthless the way you are now?	**yes**	no
13.	Do you feel full of energy?	yes	**no**
14.	Do you feel that your situation is hopeless?	**yes**	no
15.	Do you think that most people are better off than you are?	**yes**	no

A score of ≥ 5 suggests depression   **Total Score** _____

Ref. Yes average: The use of Rating Depression Series in the Elderly, in Poon (ed.): Clinical Memory Assessment of Older Adults, American Psychological Association, 1986

Fig. 1. Geriatric depression score (short form).

The Cornell Scale for Depression in Dementia (CSDD) tool is a beneficial screening tool for older adults with dementia. One aspect that makes this tool effective for older adults is that their caregivers can provide the screening tool's answers if the patient is unable. The average administration time is 30 minutes. The CSDD is the most time-consuming tool to complete. Another aspect of this screening tool's effectiveness is that it considers other health diagnoses for scoring to prevent high scores related to another diagnosis. The CSDD can protect the final score from being skewed due to the comorbidity of dementia or another disease process [17].

ANXIETY SCREENING TOOL

Ms A is a 76-year-old client who worked at her local library for 45 years before retiring 4 months ago. Ms A lives alone but has family close by. Home health services are in place due to a recent fall resulting in a fractured ankle. She is recovering well but cannot leave her home for 4 weeks. In the past, she had been very active in the community and volunteered for several organizations, but has not been able to handle this in the last several months. Most of her friends have moved away, passed away, or are unable to visit. She reports that she is very lonely and often sits and cries. Before this incidence she states that she was having trouble being in groups, worried she would get sick, and could not finish her tasks and that these symptoms are worsening with the fall. The provider decides it is in the patient's best interest to screen for anxiety using a screening tool specific to Ms A's age group. The provider decides to use the Geriatric Anxiety Inventory (GAI) screening tool.

The GAI is a validated screening tool for adults 65 years and older. The GAI is used to assess and differentiate anxiety symptoms from somatic symptoms. See Fig. 2 for the GAI, United States of America (USA-English) screening tool. See the GAI scoring instructions here: https://eshop.uniquest. com.au/gai-form-english-language-usa/. Similar to the CSDD screening tool, the GAI reduces the confusion of other medical conditions that might present with the same symptomology. Composed of 20 questions in a simple agree or disagree format, the GAI is efficient, timely, and easy to score. This tool is free for providers and persons in academia. The screening tool has been tested for both validity and reliability. However, more diverse research and use are needed in the older adult population [9,18]. One substantial issue with measuring anxiety in the population older than 65 years is the lack of construct validity, mainly due to a poor understanding of anxiety in this age group [9].

SCREENING FOLLOW-UP

When incorporating screening into practice, one obstacle to overcome is the proper steps for follow-up. Consistent, clearly thought-out actions and training with available resources will increase acceptability, screening compliance, and utilization. Much of the hesitation that surrounds screening is knowing what to do with the results of the test. Building screening tools into the electronic health record promotes efficiency for monitoring and follow-up.

GAI QUESTION

I worry a lot of the time
I find it difficult to make a decision
I often feel jumpy
I find it hard to relax
I often cannot enjoy things because of my worries
Little things bother me a lot
I often feel like I have butterflies in my stomach
I think of myself as a worrier
I can't help worrying about even trivial things
I often feel nervous
My own thoughts often make me anxious
I get an upset stomach due to my worrying
I think of myself as a nervous person
I always anticipate the worst will happen
I often feel shaky inside
I think that my worries interfere with my life
My worries often overwhelm me
I sometimes feel a great knot in my stomach
I miss out on things because I worry too much
I often feel upset

Fig. 2. Geriatric anxiety inventory—English. (*Adapted from* Pachana NA, Byrne GJ, Siddle H, Koloski N, Harley E, Arnold E. Development and validation of the Geriatric Anxiety Inventory. International Psychogeriatrics. 2007;19(1):103-114. doi:10.1017/S1041610200 6003504; with permission.)

PRACTICE SETTINGS

Screening opportunities are present in various health care settings, including home health, long-term care facilities, acute care settings, and clinics. For example, home health reaches 4.5 million clients a year with more than 12,000 agencies in the United States [19]. These home health clients could have begun or ended care at any point in 1 year [19]. Long-term care facilities have more than 1.7 million beds, with 1.3 million beds in more than 15,000 thousand facilities [20]. Eighty-two percent of adults 65 years and older are cared for by home health providers, and 84% reside in long-term care [21]. Older adults also account for about 40% of acute care admissions [22]. Clinic visits account for 498 clinic visits per year per 100 older adults [23].

Older adults residing in long-term care are at higher risk and require a more focused effort for depression screening than those in the community [24]. Various tools are available, and it is pertinent that each practice setting explores options and tools that are beneficial to their distinct needs to address mental health for older adults. Planning and incorporating a system for ensuring the correct diagnosis, treatment, and follow-up is pivotal to screening tool incorporation [13].

IMPLICATIONS FOR NURSE PRACTITIONERS

Various resources exist to assist providers with accessing the best tools. Housed on the USPSTF Web site is an app that providers can download or access via the web to examine what screening tools are most beneficial to their specific client. See Table 1 for helpful Web sites to access content. Accessing this tool can help during the planning stage choose which screening tool is most appropriate for the provider's specific clientele.

Incorporating a screening tool into one's practice has the benefit of analyzing if treatment is effective by assessing the results of the screening tool before intervention and again after an intervention has had time to exhibit a therapeutic effect [15]. Using a premodel and postmodel will assist the provider in making decisions in the care of a client and can prove beneficial in obtaining referrals or follow-up care.

The USPSTF noted risks with certain medications to treat depression in older adults. Careful consideration of comorbidities is vital in prescribing pharmacologic treatment options. Although there is a small risk, selective serotonin reuptake inhibitors increased the risk of gastrointestinal hemorrhage in clients older than 70 years [14]. There is also a risk of the syndrome of inappropriate secretion of antidiuretic hormone and hyponatremia in the older adult taking second-generation antidepressants [25]. Another helpful tool is the Beers Criteria for Potentially Inappropriate Medication Use in Older Adults. This tool provides 5 categories to assist the provider, caregiver, and client in making safe medication decisions. There are free apps and tools for both the provider and client/caregiver [26].

SUMMARY

More research is needed on translating screening tools from English to other languages [14]. Depression and anxiety screening should also be considered for caregivers of older adults. Another consideration is the lack of diversity in research using screening tools. This lack of diversity weakens the validity in certain populations [14].

Opportunities to strengthen research are present and needed, but screening remains crucial. Older adult populations are at high risk for comorbidities and poor quality of life related to anxiety and depression when left untreated [1]. With an action plan that includes screening and follow-up, these risks can be addressed and mitigated. With increased screening, opportunities to address gaps in research, such as understanding anxiety better in older adults, could be addressed.

CLINICS CARE POINTS

- Implementing depression and anxiety screening tools into practice can improve the quality of life for older adult patients.
- Having a plan in place for follow-up care is vital for a smooth transition of care and improving the mental health outcomess of older adult clients.

Acknowledgments
The author is particularly grateful for the assistance given by Dr Alyce Ashcraft and Dr Melodee Harris for their constructive feedback, useful edits, and knowledgeable recommendations.

Disclosure
I, Rebecca Clark, declare that I have no relevant or material financial interests that relate to the research described in this article.

References
[1] Centers for Disease Control and Prevention (CDC). Loneliness and social isolation linked to serious health conditions. In: Alzheimer's disease and healthy aging. 2021. Available at: https://www.cdc.gov/aging/publications/features/lonely-older-adults.html 2021. Accessed August 24, 2021.

[2] American Psychiatric Nurses Association (APNA). Whole health begins with mental health. 2021. Available at: https://www.apna.org/news/mental-health-policy/. Accessed August 23, 2021.

[3] Gerlach L, Singe SD, Kirch KM, et al. Mental health among older adults before and during the COVID-19 pandemic national poll on healthy aging. University of Michigan (Ann Arbor); 2021. Available at: www.healthyagingpoll.org/report/mental-health-among-older-adults-and-during-covid-19-pandemic. Accessed June 12, 2021.

[4] Rossom RC, Simon GE, Coleman KJ, et al. Are wishes for death or suicidal ideation symptoms of depression in older adults? Aging Ment Health 2019; https://doi.org/10.1080/13607863.2017.1423032. Available at.

[5] Centers for Disease Control and Prevention and National Association of Chronic Disease Directors. Issue brief 1 and 2. In: The State of Mental Health and Aging in America. 2021. Available at: https://www.cdc.gov/aging/publications/mental-health.html 2021. Accessed June 10, 2021.

[6] Terlizzi EP, Villarroel MA. Symptoms of generalized anxiety disorder among adults: United States, 2019. Hyattsville (MD): NCHS Data Brief, No. 378, Centers for Disease Control and Prevention. National Center for Health Statistics; 2020. Available at: https://www.cdc.gov/nchs/products/databriefs/db378.htm. Accessed July 11, 2021.

[7] Truschel J. Depression definition and DSM-5 diagnostic criteria. New York: Remedy Health Media, Psycom.net; 2020. Available at: https://www.psycom.net/depression-definition-dsm-5-diagnostic-criteria/. Accessed June 8, 2021.

[8] Reynolds CW, Kamphaus RK. BASC 3 generalized anxiety disorder 300.2 (F41.1). Pearson; 2021. Available at: https://images.pearsonclinical.com/images/assets/basc-3/basc3resources/DSM5_DiagnosticCriteria_GeneralizedAnxietyDisorder.pdfhttp://www.vin.com/Members/Proceedings/. Accessed June 5, 2021.

[9] Geriatric anxiety inventory. Why the GAI?. Available at: http://gai.net.au/. Accessed July 6, 2021.

[10] del Vecchio P. First national older adults Mental Health Awareness Day: it's about time. Rockville (MD): SAMHSA; 2018. Available at: www://blog.samhsa.gov/2018/05/17/first-national-older-adults-mental-health-awareness-day-its-about-time. Accessed June 10, 2021.

[11] Mental Health America Staff. Depression in older adults. Alexandria (VA): Mental Health America; 2021. Available at: https://mhanational.org/depression-older-adults-more-facts. Accessed June 10, 2021.

[12] Krishnamoorthy Y, Rajaa S, Rehman T. Diagnostic accuracy of various forms of geriatric depression scale for screening of depression among older adults: systematic review and meta-analysis. Arch Gerontol Geriatr 2020;87:104002. www://doi.org/10.1016/j.archger.2019.104002.

[13] Mulvaney-Day N, Marshall T, Downey Piscopo K, et al. Screening for behavioral health conditions in primary care settings: a systematic review of the literature. J Gen Intern Med 2018;. http://doi:10.1007/s11606-017-4181-0.

[14] U. S. Preventive Services Task Force (USPSTF). Prevention task force. Depression in adults screening. Available at: https://www.uspreventiveservicestaskforce.org/webview/#!/recommendation/315. Accessed on June 25, 2021.

[15] Greenberg S. The geriatric depression scale (GDS). In: Try this: best practices in care to older adults. From the hartford institute for geriatric nursing. New York University Rory Meyers College of Nursing; 2019. Available at: https://hign.org/consultgeri/try-this-series/geriatric-depression-scale-gds. Accessed on July 3, 2021.

[16] American Psychological Association. Patient Health Questionnaire (PHQ-9 & PHQ-2). 2021. Available at: https://www.apa.org/pi/about/publications/caregivers/practice-settings/assessment/tools/patient-health. Accessed July 3, 2021.

[17] Geropyschiatric Education Program. Vancouver Coastal Health. Screening tool: cornell scale for depression in dementia. Available at: https://cgatoolkit.ca/Uploads/ContentDocuments/cornell_scale_depression.pdf. Accessed July 3, 2021.

[18] American Psychological Association (APA). General anxiety inventory (GAI). 2021. Available at: https://www.apa.org/pi/about/publications/caregivers/practice-settings/assessment/tools/geriatric-anxiety. Accessed on July 3, 2021.

[19] Centers for Disease Control and Prevention (CDC). Home health statistics. 2016. Available at: https://www.cdc.gov/nchs/fastats/home-health-care.htm. Accessed June 8, 2021.

[20] Centers for Disease Control and Prevention. National Center for Health Statistics. Nursing Home Care; 2021. Available at: https://cdc.gov/nchs/fastats/nursing-home-care.htm. Accessed June 8, 2021.

[21] Centers for Disease Control and Prevention. Older persons' health. National Center for Health Statistics; 2021. Available at: https://cdc.gov/nchs/fastats/older-american-health.htm. Accessed June 10, 2021.

[22] Mattison M. Hospital management of older adults. UptoDate.com; 2021. Available at: http://uptodate.com/contents/hospital-management-of-older-adults. Accessed June 9, 2021.

[23] Ashman J, Rui P, Okeyode T. Characteristics of office-based Physician visits, 2016: NCHS data brief. 2019. Centers for Disease Control and Prevention, National Center for Health Statistics; 2019. Available at: https://cdc.gov/nchs/products/databriefs/db331.htm. Accessed June 9. 2021.

[24] Figueiredo-Duarte C, Espirito-Santo H, Sério C, et al. Validity and reliability of a shorter version of the Geriatric Depression Scale in institutionalized older Portuguese adults. Aging Mental Health 2021; https://doi.org/10.1080/13607863.2019.1695739.

[25] Gandhi S, Shariff SZ, Al-Jaishi A, et al. Second-Generation antidepressants and hyponatremia risk: a population-based cohort study of older adults. Am J Kidney Dis 2017; https://doi.org/10.1053/j.ajkd.2016.08.020.

[26] American Geriatrics Society (AGS). For older people, medications are common; updated AGS beers criteria aims to make sure they're appropriate, too. 2019. Available at: https://www.americangeriatrics.org/media-center/news/older-people-medications-are-common-updated-ags-beers-criterior-aims-make-sure. Accessed on August 24, 2021.

The Surprising Effects of Social Isolation and Loneliness on Physical Health in Older Adults

Pamela J. LaBorde, DNP, APRN, CCNS, TTSClinical Assistant Professor[a],*,
Vallon Williams, DNP, APRN, AGNP-CClinical Research Nurse Practitioner[b]

[a]University of Arkansas for Medical Sciences, College of Nursing, 4301 W Markham Street, Slot 529, Little Rock, AR 72205-7199, USA; [b]University of Arkansas for Medical Sciences, Translational Research Institute, 4301 W. Markham St., Slot 577, Little Rock, AR 72205

Keywords

- Social isolation • Loneliness • Physical health impact • Advanced practice nurse
- Health care utilization

Key points

- Social isolation and loneliness are identifiable risk factors impacting physical health outcomes.
- Understanding the impact of social isolation and loneliness on older adults' physical health facilitates health care providers' efforts to identify, prevent, and decrease adverse physical health outcomes.
- Appropriate use of assessment tools is integral to identifying loneliness and social isolation of older adults.
- Understanding the associations between social isolation, loneliness, and health care utilization will help health systems and providers examine the root causes of mental health conditions and create strategies to mitigate the consequences and need for increased health care services.
- The APRN role impacts social isolation and loneliness through education, assessment, transitional care, and public advocacy.

*Corresponding author. E-mail addresses: labordepamelaj@uams.edu (P.J.L.); vwilliams@uams.edu (V.W.)

https://doi.org/10.1016/j.yfpn.2021.12.001
2589-420X/22/

INTRODUCTION

Mental health has substantial effects on physical health and is associated with the ability to make positive, healthy lifestyle choices and participate in social engagement [1–3]. The coexistence of a mental illness and a chronic physical condition heightens the risk of poorer health outcomes. The burden of disease is attributed to lifestyle choices, especially in the older population [4,5]. Social interaction influences the adoption of healthy behaviors in decision making, access to quality health care, and support from others regarding health care decisions [1–3,5]. Two mental health issues impacting physical health are social isolation and loneliness. Social isolation is an objective consequence of few social relationships or scarce social contact, which significantly affects older adults. Social isolation is an underappreciated health risk [6]. Often, loneliness (the subjective perception of isolation) is studied and intertwined in social isolation research. Both are risk factors impacting physical health outcomes and are associated with predicting all-cause morbidity and mortality for specific physical conditions [7–9].

Social connections promote human survival. Compared with other populations, older adults tend to experience more loneliness and social isolation [10–12]. The coronavirus disease 2019 (COVID-19) pandemic created a struggle between balancing measures to prevent virus spread and the needed sacrifices to limit or curtail social connections, especially in long-term care (LTC) facilities. Social isolation and loneliness has always been a concern for those living alone or in an LTC. The pandemic heighted the impact of these preexisting threats often found in older adult populations. Psychosocial and emotional aspects rise to the top when considering the detrimental effects of social isolation and loneliness. However, there are surprising effects of social isolation and loneliness on physical health in older adults. Social isolation is a risk for premature mortality comparable to those who are obese, who smoke, or have hypertension [6,8,13].

Social isolation is prevalent in the older population due to limited financial or social resources, their social determinants of health, changes in social contacts due to deaths in family and friend circles, or changes in mobility or cognitive function [8]. About 35% of adults aged older than 45 years report loneliness [14] and 24% of adults aged older than 65 years living in community facilities report social isolation [15]. Social isolation can be intermittent or progress to a lingering condition. There are substantial mixed-gender differences in the correlation between social isolation and physical health [8]. These variances exist because men and women experience loneliness differently [8].

Gaining a better understanding of the potential for social isolation to impact the physical health of older adults facilitates efforts by health care providers (HCPs) to identify, prevent, and decrease adverse physical health outcomes. This article highlights the physical impact and 3 physical systems affected by social isolation and loneliness in older adults. In addition, information is provided on assessment, appropriate preventive interventions, the impact on health care utilization, and the role of the advanced practice registered nurse (APRN) in addressing social isolation and loneliness in older adults.

Physical health impact

The effect of depression on physical health includes alterations in cardiovascular (CV) measures such as heart rate and blood pressure and increased inflammatory responses [1,3]. Similarly, social isolation has been linked to those same conditions, as well as linked to cancer, functional decline, sleep deprivation, pain response, and sensory impairment [13,14,16]. This article discusses the impact of social isolation and loneliness on the CV, neurologic, and immune/inflammatory systems.

Cardiovascular impact

Social connectedness (specifically loneliness and social isolation) affects cardiovascular disease (CVD) development [7,8,17,18]. The results of one review showed that 72% of CV studies investigated the impact of social isolation on CV health [8]. In the context of CVD impact, the same focus for addressing CVD risk factors (biological, psychosocial, behavioral) can be applied when associating social isolation's effect on CVD [7]. However, there is insufficient evidence to support social isolation or loneliness as the *cause* of CVD. Instead, it is a *risk factor* for CVD. For example, older adults who live alone may not have available resources to access health care for an acute CV event [19]. Older adults may be more inactive, which could also lead to CVD [20].

There is a 29% increase in risk for CVD associated with few social relationships [18]. Social relationships promote lifestyle choices and encourage adherence to prescribed medical treatment plans. Social isolation results in physical inactivity and poor sleep quality, both risk factors for CVD [7]. Noted hypertension (HTN) and atherosclerosis have been associated with social isolation and loneliness [7,20,21].

Neurologic/neurovascular impact

Social relationships play a role on brain biology and reducing the incidence of stroke or cognitive decline, such as dementia [22,23]. The causation of social isolation and loneliness on neurologic mechanisms and mortality is problematic because there is limited human subject research. Animal research has been implemented to identify causal effects of social isolation on neurologic and cognitive deficits.

Social isolation and loneliness have an impact on the brain's morphology. Brain size is not directly affected by social isolation as a whole but does affect the brain regions responsible for addressing the pressures associated with socialization [23]. Maintaining a healthy physical and mental lifestyle is the best defense in protecting the aging brain and is a preventive measure against cerebrovascular disease development [24]. An inactive cognitive lifestyle, often seen in social isolation and loneliness, is linked to cognitive disorders such as dementia [25]. Bzdok and Dunbar [26] found no long-lasting adverse outcomes with short bouts of loneliness. However, continued stints of loneliness were associated with mental health (depression) and neurologic diseases (Alzheimer disease). In addition, loneliness can cause altered sleeping habits, leading to poor physical health outcomes. Neural remodeling in the dopaminergic pathway was observed in primates who were socially deprived versus those who were socially stimulated [26]. This pathway is responsible for executive functioning, reward responses, and motor function. Dysfunction with dopamine transmission has been associated with various nervous system diseases in humans [27]. Neuroremodeling in the nonhuman primates closely mimicked clinically relevant findings of those with a substance abuse disorder [26].

There is an association between social relationships and risk for stroke development. One meta-analysis found a 32% increase in risk for stroke in those who were socially isolated [18]. Another meta-analysis and systematic review [20] showed 3002 recorded stroke events from the 23 included studies and an average relative risk (1.32; 95% confidence interval 1.04, 1.68) of stroke incidence. The increased risk was attributed to exacerbations of psychosocial risk factors (increased smoking, noted depression, social disengagement, reduced physical activity) and CVD risk factors (HTN, obesity, diabetes). It is imperative to assess and address social isolation and loneliness to prevent stroke incidence.

Immune/inflammatory system impact

Loneliness and social isolation increase inflammatory response to stressors [8,21,28–30]. Communication between the brain and immune system occur through the autonomic nervous system and its 2 branches, the sympathetic nervous system (SNS) and the parasympathetic nervous system (PSNS). The fight or flight reaction of the SNS and the slowing of the immune response of the PSNS play a key role in changes to the immune system as it relates to socialization. Chronic stress associated with social isolation may result in irreversible damage to inflammatory processes [30]. Other inflammatory and immune responses impacted by social isolation and loneliness include altered cortisol responsivity [21], elevated cortisol and lowered C-reactive protein levels [8,21,28], increased proinflammatory cytokines [7,21,29], and reduced stimulation and activity of natural killer cells [21,26].

Loneliness and social disconnection increases subsequent bacterial infections, activating proinflammatory cytokines and antibacterial pathways. This increase in the risk of bacterial infections is speculated to be caused by a lack of external support or involvement in a socially hostile environment [28,31]. Human resilience is linked to social connections and social engagement. D'Acquisto [32] summarized several article reviews that described the symbiotic relationship of suffering from mental disorders with increased susceptibility to immune diseases, and vice versa.

Evidence shows that social isolation and loneliness impact physical health and psychological well-being. Efforts to mitigate the effects that social isolation and loneliness have on physical health are imperative. These efforts begin with appropriate assessment and intervention plans and understanding an APRN's role in addressing social isolation and loneliness, particularly in the older population.

HEALTH CARE ASSESSMENTS

Assessment tools are crucial to identifying loneliness and social isolation of older adults. Health care professionals use these tools to identify social isolation and loneliness singularly or combined. Factors that determine the most appropriate instrument include the purpose of the assessment, measurement quality, and target population [14,33,34]. The National Academies of Sciences, Engineering, and Medicine (NAS) [14] recommends the Berkman-Syme Social Network Index (SNI) to measure social isolation in the clinical environment because of its brevity, availability, and validated translations. The SNI tool evaluates social relationships based on the following factors: marriage, contacts with close friends and family, church membership, and informal and formal group associations. Each element represents one point with lower scores suggesting higher levels of isolation [35]. Marriage, close contacts, and church membership showed statistical significance relating to mortality risk [36].

The Lubben Social Network Scale (LSNS) a derivative of the Berkman-Syme SNI, is a 10-item assessment tool used to detect social isolation in older adults [14]. The 12-item LSNS-R, a revision of the LSNS, clarifies the relationship between family, friendship, and community networks [37]. The more extensive LSNS-18 is used primarily in social science research, whereas the brevity of LSNS-6 helps screen for social isolation of older adults in the clinical setting [37]. The first 3 questions of the LSNS-6 concern family connections, whereas the last 3 questions address nonfamily or friend links [38]. The LSNS-6 has high internal consistency ($\alpha = 0.83$) and a consistent factor structure [38]. The total weight of the LSNS-6 is 30, and a score less than 12 indicates an increased risk for social isolation [38].

The Revised University of California Los Angeles Loneliness Scale (R-UCLA) includes 20 self-administered questions and measures subjective loneliness [14]. R-UCLS has high internal consistency with significant discriminant validity "against measures of personality, social desirability, and depression" [39]. The combined weight of the tool is 80, with higher scores pointing to a greater level of loneliness [40,41].

The Three Item Loneliness Scale (3ILS) adapts the R-UCLA and lends itself to the clinical environment due to its conciseness. Hughes and colleagues [41] report adequate reliability with convergent and discriminant validity. Older adults are the target population for the 3ILS, making it more advantageous for assessing loneliness in this demographic [41]. Furthermore, the NAS [14] recommends the clinical use of this tool to measure loneliness in older adults.

INTERVENTIONS

Assessment results indicating increased loneliness or social isolation require interventions to improve outcomes. Four ways to classify interventions to reduce social isolation and loneliness are to hone social skills, improve social skills, grow social interactions, and tackle maladaptive social cognition [33]. Friendly visitors, meal delivery programs, and in-home support groups are examples of interventions to improve social skills [42]. Increased access to social interactions may involve telephone or online outreach, social activities, and transportation assistance. The use of social media to connect with family and others increased during the pandemic. LTC facilities tried to maintain regular scheduling of activities deemed pleasurable for older adults (exercise programs, music therapy, mindfulness programs, and so forth) individually. Using the television or YouTube channels can help provide such programs. Another way to improve access to social interaction is to provide assistive devices to enhance functional ability, such as eyeglasses to improve vision, hearing aids to help with listening, and walking aids to assist with mobility [42].

Interventions used to help improve social skills and address maladaptive social cognition may include mindfulness and psychotherapy. Mindfulness is awareness of the present time with intent and without judgment [43]. One randomized controlled study showed that the Mindfulness-Based Stress Reduction (MBSR) program helped reduce loneliness in older adults versus an increase in loneliness in the control group [44,45]. The MBSR intervention successfully decreased HTN and nonmotor Parkinson symptoms like anxiety, depression, and stress in prior research [43]. Interpersonal psychotherapy and cognitive-behavioral therapy (CBT) interventions also help improve social skills and address maladaptive social cognition. Interpersonal therapy focuses on incongruent thoughts concerning interpersonal relationships, and CBT helps to transform obstructive social perceptions [14,42].

Intervention methods vary based on environment, delivery modality, and treatment goals. Support groups can enhance social engagement and increase social interactions by directly focusing on social isolation and loneliness or at a particular activity in a group setting that promotes social interactions [14]. Technological interventions such as video gaming and computer utilization education help improve social isolation and loneliness in older persons. It is essential to evaluate whether an increase in technology-based socialization may increase loneliness rates due to decreased time spent with others when considering technological-based interventions [33]. See Table 1 for categories of interventions.

HEALTH CARE UTILIZATION

Research has evolved regarding the impact that social isolation and loneliness have on health care utilization. Earlier studies applied the Andersen Behavioral Model, which theorizes that 4 factors influence health care utilization:

1. Environment (health care system and person's external environment)
2. Population characteristics (predisposing conditions, resource utilization, individual needs)
3. Health behavior (health services used, health practices)
4. Outcomes (perception of personal health status, satisfaction with services received) [46].

Table 1
Categories of interventions to prevent social isolation and loneliness[a]

Category	Intervention
Social facilitation interventions	• Group-based activities (clubs, shared interest topic groups, senior day care centers, friendship enrichment programs) • Technology-based solutions (videoconferencing with family & friends, social networking)
Psychological therapies	• Humor & laughter therapy • Mindfulness & stress reduction • Reminiscence group therapy • Cognitive & social support interventions
Health & social care provision	• Formal care programs in long-term care facilities or community settings • CARELINK program (http://doi:10.3928/19404921-20130110-01) • Eden alternative model (https://www.edenalt.org)
Animal interventions	• Individual settings • Live dog/cat vs robotic dog/cat • Pet therapy
Befriending interventions	• One-to-one intervention with volunteers • Aims to support the lonely individual • Senior Companion Program • Call in Time program (https://www.ageuk.org.uk/wigan-borough/our-services/call-in-time/)
Leisure/skill development interventions	• Gardening programs • Computer/Internet use • Volunteer work • Holiday activities • Sport activities • Engaging in hobbies • Reading/watching television

[a]*Interventions to reduce social isolation and loneliness among older people: An integrative review.*
Data from Gardiner C, Geldenhuys G, Gott M. Interventions to reduce social isolation and loneliness among older people: an integrative review. Health Soc Care Community. 2018;26(2):147–157. https://doi.org/10.1111/hsc.12367.

More recent studies have investigated health care utilization in different realms such as financial burden, hospital admissions, emergency department (ED) visits, and utilization of outpatient services. There is an additional $6.7 million output in Medicare payments due to social isolation [47]. Compared with widowed older adults who are not socially isolated, there is an increase of $3,276 individual Medicare spending in those who were socially isolated [48,49]. Medicare spent an additional $153 for beneficiaries who were deemed as lonely, compared with those who were not lonely [49]. Although loneliness has been linked to an increase in Medicare spending, spending for the lonely is lower than the expenditures for those experiencing objective social isolation [49].

Results from a retrospective, observational study assessing the relationship between social isolation and ED utilization and hospital admissions utilization noted that individuals who reported feeling socially isolated *sometimes* were more likely to have at least one hospital admission. Those who experienced social isolation *sometimes* or *often/always* were more likely to have at least one ED visit [50]. HCPs should consider self-reported social isolation to predict future hospital admissions and ED utilization.

Valtorta and colleagues [51] showed robust linkage evidence between social relationships and early hospital readmissions and moderate evidence indicating an association between smaller social networks and increased length of hospital stays. However, there was inadequate evidence to establish that older adults with more fragile social ties overutilize ambulatory care that exceeds their needs. Broader social networks depend on outpatient services more than persons with reduced social ties [14]. For example, older adults who lack social support such as adequate transportation may underutilize health care systems due to impaired access to care [52]. The onset of the COVID-19 pandemic created more barriers for older adults seeking ambulatory care who had fewer social relations. Wong and colleagues [53] reported older adult primary care patients with multiple chronic health conditions experienced deteriorating psychosocial health and had more missed scheduled medical visits during the start of the COVID-19 outbreak. The pandemic caused an abrupt interruption in these visits through elective procedure moratoriums, suspension of outpatient visits, and increased use of telehealth medicine in place of in-person medical visits [54].

Understanding the associations between social isolation, loneliness, and health care utilization will help health systems and HCPs examine the root causes of loneliness and social isolation and implement strategies to mitigate the consequences and need for increased health care services. These strategies aim to improve health outcomes by using cost-effective health care system interventions and resources. HCPs can implement strategies to address the social risks of social isolation and loneliness. Examples include

- consistent screenings and assessments for social isolation and loneliness,
- collaborating with community resources to help connect individuals with opportunities for social engagement,
- incorporating services such as case management to address care coordination, and
- referrals to community resources [48,49].

ADVANCE PRACTICE REGISTERED NURSE ROLE

The APRN role impacts social isolation and loneliness in the aging demographic through education, assessments, transitional care, and public advocacy. One of the first tasks of the APRN evaluating loneliness and social isolation in older adults is to conduct a health history that includes a thorough personal and social history (Box 1) [55]. Additional components of the psychosocial assessment should consist of screening for dementia, anxiety, sleep habits, and functional status. The APRN must develop a care plan that provides appropriate interventions and follow-up for older adults experiencing social isolation and loneliness.

Box 1: Components of personal and social history[a]

- Personality and interests
- Sources of support
- Coping style
- Strengths and concerns
- Occupation
- Education
- Military service
- Job history
- Financial situation
- Retirement

- Significant others
- Religious preference
- Spiritual beliefs
- ADL
- IADL
- Physical activity
- Healthy nutrition
- Safety measures
- Sexual orientation and practices
- Transportation source

Abbreviations: ADL, activities of daily living; IADL, instrumental activities of daily living.
[a]Bates' guide to physical examination and history taking.

Data from Bickley LS, Szilagyi PG, Bates B. Bates' guide to physical examination and history taking. 12th ed. Philadelphia: Wolters Kluwer; 2017.

Combatting social isolation and loneliness in older adults does not stop with identification and assessment. The APRN addresses the patient's physical needs and is aware of the possible impact of social isolation and loneliness on physical health if noted during screening. The APRN can provide transitional care by making necessary referrals to help address social, sensory, physical rehabilitation, and other needs.

The APRN's role extends to promoting public health advocacy concerning social isolation and loneliness in aging persons at a community level. Social cohesion, which is companionship and the notion of community solidarity, is one of the critical issues of the Social and Community Context domain of Healthy People 2030 [56]. There is a risk for reduced social cohesion in the older population because social interactions with friends decline with aging [56]. Social prescribing is one method to help promote social cohesion in aging adults. Social prescribing is a community-based therapy initiated by the HCP to connect patients with community supports tailored to their needs [57]. Examples can involve activities such as community gardening or trips to the art gallery. Social prescribing helps navigate older adults experiencing social isolation and loneliness to programs that assist with benefits, bereavement support, creative arts, neighborhood gardening, employment advice, health behavior, or housing [57]. However, social prescribing and its potential benefits warrant more research to help establish efficacy and implementation [58].

IMPLICATIONS FOR PRACTICE

The concepts and measures discussed need to be a part of primary, secondary, and tertiary prevention endeavors initiated by HCPs, such as APRNs. The health care system cannot act alone in addressing social isolation and loneliness among older adults. The health care system can play an integral part in reducing the risks of experiencing adverse physical health effects through assessments, screenings, and the formation of individualized plans of care, which include referrals to appropriate resources [14]. Further research is needed to enrich and strengthen evidence-based information and strategies to prevent social isolation and loneliness.

SUMMARY

Loneliness and social isolation are social determinant risk factors impacting physical health. When humans experience social isolation, their brain functions self-protectively, affecting behavioral, mental, and physical health. If allowed to continue for long periods, the consequences can affect mortality and the development and progression of chronic diseases into the later years of life. Social isolation and loneliness may be underappreciated public health concerns. Public health initiatives that focus on promoting social connections as a priority facilitate preventive measures. Heightening the awareness of social isolation and loneliness' surprising impacts on physical health will effectively improve HCP's efforts to care for persons experiencing these mental health concerns. Doing so would benefit overall public health and well-being.

CLINICS CARE POINTS

- Consistent social isolation and loneliness screening is an integral component of preventive care for older adults. The LSNS-6 (social isolation) and 3ILS (loneliness) are beneficial in the clinical setting due to their brevity.
- Consider lifestyle, financial security, transportation, sensory impairments, access to technology, and other social determinants of health when establishing interventions to improve social isolation and loneliness.
- Potential referrals to address barriers to social engagement include audiology, ophthalmology, and rehabilitation services.

Disclosure

Authors have nothing to disclose.

References

[1] Ahmedani BK, Peterson EL, Young H, et al. Major physical health conditions and risk of suicide. Am J Prev Med 2017;53(3):308–15.
[2] Ohrnberger J, Fichera E, Sutton M. The relationship between physical and mental health: A mediation analysis. Soc Sci Med 2017;195:42–9.
[3] National Institute of Mental Health. Chronic illness and mental health: recognizing and treating depression. Bethesda, MD: National Institute of Health; 2021. Available at: https://www.nimh.nih.gov/health/publications/chronic-illness-mental-health/. Accessed July 08, 2021.
[4] World Health Organization. Global health risks: mortality and burden of disease attributable to selected major risks. Geneva, Switzerland: World Health Organization; 2009.

Available at: https://www.who.int/healthinfo/global_burden_disease/GlobalHealthRisks_report_full.pdf. Accessed August 04, 2021.

[5] Melzer D, Tavakoly B, Winder R, et al. Health care quality for an active later life: improving quality of prevention and treatment through information - England 2005 to 2012. Peninsula College of Medicine and Dentistry Ageing Research Group for Age UK. Exeter, UK: University of Exeter; 2012. Accessed August 04, 2021.

[6] Simard J, Volicer L. Loneliness and isolation in long-term care and the COVID-19 pandemic. J Am Med Directors Assoc 2020;21(7):966–7.

[7] Xia N, Li H. Loneliness, social isolation, and cardiovascular health. Antioxid Redox Signal 2018;28(9):837–51.

[8] Courtin E, Knapp M. Social isolation, loneliness and health in old age: A scoping review. Health Soc Care Community 2017;25(3):799–812.

[9] Landeiro F, Barrows P, Musson EN, et al. Reducing social isolation and loneliness in older people: a systematic review protocol. BMJ Open 2017;7:e013778.

[10] Iliffe S, Kharicha K, Harari D, et al. Health risk appraisal in older people 2: the implications for clinicians and commissioners of social isolation risk in older people. Br J Gen Pract 2007;57(537):277–82.

[11] Shankar A, McMunn A, Banks J, et al. Loneliness, social isolation, and behavioral and biological health indicators in older adults. Health Psychol 2011;30(4):377–85.

[12] Theeke LA. Predictors of loneliness in U.S. adults over age sixty-five. Arch Psychiatr Nurs 2009;23(5):387–96.

[13] Leaman MC, Azios JH. Experiences of social distancing during coronavirus disease 2019 as a catalyst for changing long-term care culture. Am J Speech Lang Pathol 2021;30(1): 318–23.

[14] National Academies of Sciences, Engineering, and Medicine. Social isolation and loneliness in older adults: opportunities for the health care system. Washington DC: National Academies Press; 2020; https://doi.org/10.17226/25663.

[15] Cudjoe TKM, Roth DL, Szanton SL, et al. The Epidemiology of Social Isolation: National Health and Aging Trends Study. J Gerontol B Psychol Sci Soc Sci 2020;75(1):107–13.

[16] Bethell J, Aelick K, Babineau J, et al. Social connection in long-term care homes: A scoping review of published research on the mental health impacts and potential strategies during COVID-19. J Am Med Directors Assoc 2021;22(2):228.

[17] Holt-Lunstad J, Smith TB, Baker M, et al. Loneliness and social isolation as risk factors for mortality: A meta-analytic review. Perspect Psychol Sci 2015;10(2):227–37.

[18] Bu F, Steptoe A, Fancourt D. Relationship between loneliness, social isolation and modifiable risk factors for cardiovascular disease: A latent class analysis. J Epidemiol Community Health 2021;75:749–54.

[19] Smith RW, Barnes I, Green J, et al. Social isolation and risk of heart disease and stroke: analysis of two large UK prospective studies. Lancet Public Health 2021;6(4):e232–9.

[20] Valtorta NK, Kanaan M, Gilbody S, et al. Loneliness and social isolation as risk factors for coronary heart disease and stroke: Systematic review and meta-analysis of longitudinal observational studies. Heart 2016;102(13):1009–16.

[21] Hackett RA, Hamer M, Endrighi R, et al. Loneliness and stress-related inflammatory and neuroendocrine responses in older men and women. Psychoneuroendocrinology 2012;37(11):1801–9.

[22] Mohammed AH, Zhu SW, Darmopil S, et al. Environmental enrichment and the brain. Prog In Brain Res 2002;138:109–33.

[23] Cacioppo S, Capitanio JP, Cacioppo JT. Toward a neurology of loneliness. Psychol Bull 2014;140(6):1464–504.

[24] Peters R. Ageing and the brain. Postgrad Med J 2006;82(964):84–8.

[25] Valenzuela MJ, Matthews FE, Brayne C, et al. Multiple biological pathways link cognitive lifestyle to protection from dementia. Soc Biol Psychiatry 2012;71(9):783–91.

[26] Bzdok D, Dunbar RIM. The neurobiology of social distance. Trends Cogn Sci 2020;24(9): 717–33.

[27] Juárez Olguín H, Calderón Guzmán D, Hernández García E, et al. The role of dopamine and its dysfunction as a consequence of oxidative stress. Oxidative Med Cell Longevity 2016;2016:9730467.

[28] Hawkley LC, Capitanio JP. Perceived social isolation, evolutionary fitness and health outcomes: a lifespan approach. Philosophical Trans R Soc 2015;370(1669):20140114.

[29] Moieni M, Irwin MR, Jevtic I, et al. Trait sensitivity to social disconnection enhances pro-inflammatory responses to a randomized controlled trial of endotoxin. Psychoneuroendocrinology 2015;62:336–42.

[30] Friedler B, Crapser J, McCullough L. One is the deadliest number: the detrimental effects of social isolation on cerebrovascular diseases and cognition. Acta Neuropathol 2015;129(4):493–509.

[31] Lasselin J, Alvarez-Salas E, Grigoleit JS. Well-being and immune response: a multi-system perspective. Curr Opin Pharmacol 2016;29:34–41.

[32] D'Acquisto F. Affective immunology: where emotions and the immune response converge. Dialogues Clin Neurosci 2017;19(1):9–19.

[33] Perissinotto C, Holt-Lunstad J, Periyakoil VS, et al. A practical approach to assessing and mitigating loneliness and isolation in older adults. J Am Geriatr Soc 2019;67(4):657–62.

[34] Berkman LF, Syme SL. Social networks, host resistance, and mortality: A nine-year follow-up study of Alameda County residents. Am J Epidemiol 2017;185(11):1070–88.

[35] Hamilton CM, Strader LC, Pratt JG, et al. The PhenX Toolkit: Get the most from your measures. Am J Epidemiol 2011;174(3):253–60.

[36] Berkman LF, Breslow L. Health and ways on living: the alameda county study. New York: Oxford University Press; 1983.

[37] Boston College. Description of the LSNS. Available at: https://www.bc.edu/bc-web/schools/ssw/sites/lubben/description.html. Accessed July 08, 2021.

[38] Lubben J, Blozik E, Gillmann G, et al. Performance of an abbreviated version of the Lubben Social Network Scale among three European community-dwelling older adult populations. Gerontologist 2006;46(4):503–13.

[39] Russell DW. UCLA Loneliness Scale (Version 3): Reliability, validity, and factor structure. J Pers Assess 1996;66(1):20–40.

[40] Russell D, Peplau LA, Cutrona CE. The revised UCLA Loneliness Scale: Concurrent and discriminant validity evidence. J Pers Soc Psychol 1980;39(3):472–80.

[41] Hughes ME, Waite LJ, Hawkley LC, et al. A short scale for measuring loneliness in large surveys: Results from two population-based studies. Res Aging 2004;26(6):655–72.

[42] Education Development Center. Reducing loneliness and social isolation among older adults. Suicide Prevention Resource Center 2020. Available at: https://sprc.org/sites/default/files/Reducing%20Loneliness%20and%20Social%20Isolation%20Among%20Older%20Adults%20Final.pdf. Accessed July 08, 2021.

[43] Felsted KF. Mindfulness, stress, and aging. Clin Geriatr Med 2020;36(4):685–96.

[44] Creswell JD, Irwin MR, Burklund LJ, et al. Mindfulness-Based Stress Reduction training reduces loneliness and pro-inflammatory gene expression in older adults: A small randomized controlled trial. Brain Behav Immun 2012;26(7):1095–101.

[45] Gardiner C, Geldenhuys G, Gott M. Interventions to reduce social isolation and loneliness among older people: an integrative review. Health Soc Care Community 2018;26(2): 147–57.

[46] Andersen RM. Revisiting the behavioral model and access to medical care: Does it matter? J Health Soc Behav 1995;36(1):1–10.

[47] Flowers L, House A, Noel-Miller C, et al. Medicare spends more on socially isolated older adults. Washington DC: AARP Public Policy Institute; 2017. Available at: https://www.aarp.org/content/dam/aarp/ppi/2017/10/medicare-spends-more-on-socially-isolated-older-adults.pdf. Accessed July 14, 2021.

[48] Bhatt J, McKinney J. Social isolation and loneliness are America's next public health issue. Chicago, IL: Becker's Healthc; 2019. Available at: https://www.beckershospitalreview.com/care-coordination/social-isolation-and-loneliness-are-america-s-next-public-health-issue.html. Accessed July 14, 2021.

[49] Shaw JG, Farid M, Noel-Miller C, et al. Social isolation and medicare spending: among older adults, objective social isolation increases expenditures while loneliness does not. J Aging Health 2017;29(7):1119–43.

[50] Mosen DM, Banegas MP, Tucker-Seeley RD, et al. Social isolation associated with future health care utilization. Popul Health Management 2021;24(3):333–7.

[51] Valtorta NK, Moore DC, Barron L, et al. Older adults' social relationships and health care utilization: a systematic review. Am J Public Health 2018;108(4):e1–10.

[52] Elder K, Retrum J. Framework for isolation in adults over 50. Long Beach, CA: AARP Foundation; 2012. Available at: https://www.aarp.org/content/dam/aarp/aarp_foundation/2012_PDFs/AARP-Foundation-Isolation-Framework-Report.pdf. Accessed July 08, 2021.

[53] Wong SYS, Zhang D, Sit RWS, et al. Impact of COVID-19 on loneliness, mental health, and health service utilisation: A prospective cohort study of older adults with multimorbidity in primary care. Br J Gen Pract 2020;70(700):e817–24.

[54] Anderson KE, McGinty EE, Presskreischer R, et al. Reports of forgone medical care among US adults during the initial phase of the COVID-19 pandemic. JAMA Netw Open 2021;4(1):1–11.

[55] Bickley LS, Szilagyi PG, Bates B. Bates' Guide to physical examination and history taking. 12th edition. Philadelphia (PA): Wolters Kluwer; 2017.

[56] Office of Disease Prevention and Health Promotion. Social cohesion. U.S. Department of Health and Human Services. Available at: https://health.gov/healthypeople/objectives-and-data/social-determinants-health/literature-summaries/social-cohesion. Accessed July 08, 2021.

[57] Savage RD, Stall NM, Rochon PA. Looking before we leap: Building the evidence for social prescribing for lonely older adults. J Am Geriatr Soc 2020;68(2):429–31.

[58] Hamilton-West K, Milne A, Hotham S. New horizons in supporting older people's health and wellbeing: is social prescribing a way forward? Age Ageing 2020;49(3):319–26.

The Mental Health and Well Being of Older Adults in Hospice and Palliative Care

Maeghan E. Arnold, DNP, APRN, AGACNP-BC[a,b,*]

[a]College of Nursing, University of Arkansas for Medical Sciences, 4301 West Markham Street, Slot 529, Little Rock, AR 72205, USA; [b]Baptist Health Medical Center, Little Rock, AR, USA

Keywords

- Hospice • Palliative care • End of life • Older adult • Anxiety • Depression
- Quality of life

Key points

- Anxiety and depression are the most cited mental health concerns in older adults at the end of life.
- Screening tools provide subjective and objective data for clinicians to assess anxiety, depression, quality of life, and the need for palliative or hospice services.
- Palliative care and hospice care use an interdisciplinary approach to care for patients holistically (physically, emotionally, and spiritually).
- Palliative care and hospice care are not mutually exclusive; palliative care can be provided during curative treatment, while hospice care can only be provided to patients who are terminally ill (less than 6-month life expectancy).
- Patients who receive palliative care services demonstrate improved anxiety, depression, and quality of life when compared with standard care.

INTRODUCTION

There is a significant focus on physical comorbidities in older adults, but mental health is often overlooked. Risk factors for depression in older adults are often multifactorial. This may stem from chronic medical diagnoses and physical impairments that limit function as well as socialization [1]. Anxiety and depression are frequently cited in health care literature as the most

*College of Nursing, University of Arkansas for Medical Sciences, 4301 West Markham Street, Slot 529, Little Rock, AR 72205. E-mail address: MEArnold@uams.edu

https://doi.org/10.1016/j.yfpn.2022.01.001

prevalent mental health concerns of older adults with life-limiting illnesses [2,3]. Both palliative care and mental health are stigmatized in the United States, which may further impede diagnosis and treatment of anxiety and depression in older adults with chronic, life-limiting illnesses. It is imperative that health care providers (HCPs) frequently assess anxiety, depression, and quality of life (QOL) in older adults experiencing chronic illness, understand the difference between palliative care and hospice care, and provide education to patients and families to destigmatize palliative and mental health care.

CASE PRESENTATION

Ms. B is an octogenarian with significant past medical history for hypertension (HTN), diabetes mellitus type 2 (T2DM), hyperlipidemia, obesity, anemia of chronic disease, iron deficiency anemia, and chronic kidney disease (CKD). She presented to the emergency department (ED) with complaints of shortness of breath and increased bilateral lower extremity (LE) edema. At the time of presentation, she was taking furosemide in addition to her other home medications. Her chest radiograph revealed pulmonary edema; she was admitted for observation. During her stay, diuretic therapy was maximized; her kidney function had declined since her last nephrology appointment. A decision was made in the hospital to begin temporary dialysis in hopes her kidney function would improve. Upon discharge, Ms. B. began outpatient dialysis 3 times weekly. Unfortunately, her kidneys did not recover, and it was explained that she would need long-term dialysis.

After the first 6 months of Ms. B.'s dialysis, her mobility was significantly decreased because of weakness, dizziness, fatigue, and shortness of breath. Because of the COVID-19 pandemic, her ability to leave her independent living facility was greatly diminished, and meals were no longer offered in the main dining room. After each dialysis session, she experienced severe nausea and weakness. She was prescribed ondansetron for nausea that was largely ineffective. Because of nausea, she experienced poor appetite and became protein malnourished, further exacerbating her LE edema. At an HCP office visit, it was determined she had depression and was prescribed sertraline. Sertraline further exacerbated her dizziness and nausea and was subsequently discontinued. No further medications for depression were initiated after discontinuation of sertraline. As her family watched her quality of life diminish, at least 3 attempts were made to discuss palliative care and hospice for Ms. B. The family was informed that while dialysis could be discontinued at any time, her renal laboratory values and vital signs trends were stable, suggesting she was tolerating dialysis well.

Beginning with the ninth month of dialysis, Ms. B. had increased visits to the ED because of shortness of breath, chest pain, palpitations, severe headache, and/or falls. Between months 9 and 15 of dialysis, she was admitted to observation status or inpatient status 6 times. She developed atrial fibrillation, but because of high fall risk, was not started on anticoagulation. She was diagnosed with sick sinus syndrome; because of increased risk of infection and clotting, she was not eligible for a pacemaker.

Fourteen months after dialysis initiation, sessions were shortened because of hypotension and subsequently, an inability to pull off sufficient volumes. During that month, Ms. B.'s mentation declined because of uremic encephalopathy. Initially, she experienced increasing forgetfulness. She also fell and sustained a painful, inoperable pelvic ramus fracture and was admitted to the hospital. She was discharged to a rehabilitation facility for physical therapy, with plans to continue dialysis. One week after admission to the rehabilitation facility, her confusion worsened, and she was sleeping most of the day and unable to participate in therapy. Another call was made to the nephrologist who again informed the family that Ms. B.'s laboratory values remained stable. Because of increased somnolence and confusion, the decision was made by her family to transition to inpatient hospice. After 1 day of inpatient hospice care, she was comatose. She died 3 days later.

PALLIATIVE CARE

The word palliate means to "relieve or lesson without curing; mitigate; alleviate." [4] Palliative care focuses on alleviating symptoms for various chronic illnesses. Palliative care is often referred to as an additional layer of support for patients experiencing chronic illnesses. Patients receiving palliative care can continue to pursue curative measures. For example, a patient with advanced breast cancer undergoing chemotherapy and radiation treatments can receive palliative care for pain, nausea, hot flashes, depression, anxiety, insomnia, fatigue, and/or neuropathy [5]. As palliative care treats patients holistically, quality of life during aggressive treatment can be optimized, regardless of prognosis. Palliative care services, though highly stigmatized, do not mean that a patient is dying [6]. Palliative care services can be provided in hospitals, clinics, many types of living environments, or the patient's home [7]. Ideally, palliative care specialists and the primary treatment team work collaboratively to address patient symptoms. Earlier palliative care intervention has been demonstrated to improve physical symptoms, mental well-being, and quality of life [8]. In addition, referral to palliative care has demonstrated significant cost savings [9,10].

Ms. B. could have benefitted from an early palliative care referral, beginning with her diagnosis of end-stage renal disease (ESRD) and dialysis initiation. A community-based palliative care team could have visited her at her independent living facility, aggressively managed her symptoms of nausea, anorexia, fatigue, depression, and pain, all while allowing her to continue her dialysis treatments. Palliative care would have been instrumental in educating Ms. B. on advanced directives and end-of-life (EOL) planning. Initiation of a palliative care referral would have allowed a more seamless transition to hospice care when she began to experience increasing confusion and somnolence. The team could have supported the family as they made the difficult decision to transition from aggressive measures with dialysis to comfort-focused care in Ms. B.'s last days.

HOSPICE CARE

Hospice care is a type of palliative care that is provided when curative measures are no longer effective, or when the patient has experienced effects that have rendered the curative measure intolerable. Medicare guidelines stipulate patients must have documentation from 2 physicians attesting a terminal illness with 6 months or less to live if curative treatments are withheld [11]. Once this documentation has been submitted by the hospice organization, additional paperwork is signed by the patient or power of attorney (POA) agreeing to cessation of treatment for the terminal illness or related conditions [11]. This paperwork indicates that a shift has been made to comfort measures. Hospice care can be provided in various settings, including hospitals, long-term care (LTC) facilities, free-standing hospice facilities, or the patient's residence. The level of care is guided by the patient's needs [11].

Ms. B. received hospice services in a free-standing, inpatient hospice unit. Because of the abrupt decline in her health status, her family was unable to make the necessary arrangements for her to be cared for at home. If a patient lives in a private residence or an independent living facility, social support must be assessed. For patients living in LTC facilities, 24-hour care is already available. As routine home care under the Medicare Hospice Benefit relies on family or hired caregivers for day-to-day needs, home care can be challenging for relatives who are still working or lack the space for a hospital bed and other necessary equipment. Although Medicare provides weekly nursing and nursing assistant services through the Medicare Hospice Benefit, finances must be considered if additional home assistance is required, as this would be an out-of-pocket expense. If family support is abundant, it is also important to assess whether the caregiver can lift, turn, bathe, and change patients who are bedridden. Additional skills, such as dressing changes for extensive wounds, should also be considered when making a hospice referral.

CAREGIVERS

It is crucial that caregivers of patients receiving palliative and hospice care services are not forgotten. Whether a patient is receiving palliative or hospice care, a nurse generally visits the home once per week to perform an assessment, assist with medication refills, and at times, set up the medication in a pill pack. A nursing assistant may visit between 3 to 5 times per week to assist with bathing and dressing for the day. A social worker may visit occasionally, particularly when issues arise such as a need for respite care. A chaplain is available for patients who are interested. However, despite this interdisciplinary care, much of the work is left to the caregiver at home.

Patients who are combative or resistant to feeding or changing may cause frustration for the caregiver. Those who lack health care training may not understand why the patient is not cooperating. It may be difficult for caregivers to cope with the seemingly ever-changing moods of a patient with dementia or brain metastases. Patients with difficulty transferring or who are bedbound may cause increased emotional and physical fatigue due to the physically demanding work of caregiving. Perhaps a patient was once the spiritual figure-head for the family but is no longer able to say a prayer at mealtimes or lacks interest or is cognitively unable to participate in important rituals (eg, eucharist, anointing, or fasting). This can be a source of spiritual distress for the caregiver. It is difficult to watch someone decline when he or she has been viewed as a source of strength, a confidant, or one who can be sought for comfort and is no longer fulfill those roles, whether due to cognitive or physical impairment. While the literature identifies those at increased risk for caregiver role strain, there is a paucity of literature that identifies an effective means to rectify the issue. Palliative care professionals are poised to teach coping skills to caregivers, but this does not alleviate the physical stressors of caregiving. At the end of the day, the patient still needs care, and if there is aversion to long-term care or finances preclude it, the caregiver is left to do the work.

LITERATURE

Palliative care and hospice care are available for various chronic conditions, including ESRD, chronic obstructive pulmonary disease (COPD), heart failure (HF), cancer, stroke, and degenerative neurologic conditions (eg, Huntington disease, amyotrophic lateral sclerosis, Parkinson disease, Alzheimer disease, and multiple sclerosis) [12]. Palliative care and hospice care focus on aggressive symptom management in patients with chronic conditions, including mental health issues such as anxiety and depression. HCPs should be comfortable administering and interpreting results of screening tools such as the 2-item Patient Health Questionnaire (PHQ-2) or the 9-item version (PHQ-9) to aid in diagnosis of depression [13]. Additionally, the Geriatric Depression Scale (GDS) is useful when assessing elderly patients [14]. When assessing patients for anxiety, the 7-item General Anxiety Disorder Scale (GAD-7) is a reliable and validated tool [15].

Earlier intervention and consultation of palliative care have been documented throughout the literature to improve outcomes in physical manifestations of illness, psychological effects of illness, and spiritual/existential distress. A study by Greer and colleagues demonstrated that patients who received palliative care services earlier in their cancer diagnosis improved coping skills, in addition to physical, social, emotional, and functional aspects of quality of life [16]. Interdisciplinary care for palliative care patients is essential in management of patients with complex illnesses, as comorbidities of anxiety and depression are often present [17].

In addition to improved coping skills, pharmacologic management is available to patients receiving palliative care and hospice services. The American Psychological Association's Clinical Practice Guideline for Depression recommends 3 drug classes for consideration when prescribing antidepressants for older adults [18]. Second-generation selective-norepinephrine reuptake inhibitors (SSRIs), norepinephrine-dopamine reuptake inhibitors (NDRIs), and selective-norepinephrine reuptake inhibitors (SNRIs) are well-tolerated overall and have a lower risk of adverse effects [18]. Second-generation SSRIs include escitalopram, paroxetine, fluoxetine, sertraline, and citalopram. NDRIs are also called atypical antidepressants; bupropion is the primary medication sold in this category [19]. Bupropion is unique in that, unlike other antidepressants, it is not associated with weight gain or sedation [19]. SNRIs include duloxetine and venlafaxine, and are helpful in patients with neuropathic pain and depression. As with all medications in older adults, the best approach is to start low and go slow. Although pain management is beyond the scope of this article, it is important to note its association with psychological comorbidities, such as depression. Untreated or undertreated pain further exacerbates depressive symptoms and increases feelings of hopelessness, particularly in the setting of chronic and life-limiting illnesses. In addition to an SNRI, ketamine may be beneficial in the palliative care setting to target depression and pain [20,21].

Patients receiving pharmacologic therapy for anxiety should be prescribed an SSRI or an SNRI, as these medications are first-line [18]. Benzodiazepines should be avoided, particularly in the elderly. An additional medication for consideration in the treatment of anxiety is gabapentin, an anticonvulsant [18]. Like SNRIs, gabapentin is a medication with neuropathic pain benefits, and is commonly used as an adjunct in treatment of cancer pain [22].

An additional benefit of palliative care, particularly early palliative care, has been associated with decreased health care costs in older adults. A propensity score-matched retrospective cohort study by Miller and colleagues examined earlier palliative care intervention in US nursing homes and the association with health care costs, ED visits, and hospitalizations [9]. The study demonstrated significant cost savings when palliative care was consulted within the last 6 months of life, but before the last week of life [9]. In addition, there was a significant decrease in ED visits and hospitalizations for palliative care patients, which reduces health care expenditures due to unnecessary procedures and treatments [9]. A matched cohort study by Sheridan and colleagues noted a 25% decrease in cost for palliative care patients [10]. The authors also noted that with early palliative care initiation, at least 1 month prior to death, the cost savings were greater [10].

REFERRALS/RESOURCES

Most hospitals have an inpatient palliative care specialist or team that can facilitate outpatient care after discharge. However, HCP or other specialists can also initiate a referral to outpatient palliative or hospice care services based on the patient's needs and goals. Some organizations have a community-based palliative care program, home hospice, and an inpatient hospice unit to allow for transitions of care as dictated by the patient's evolving care needs. The National Hospice and Palliative Care Organization (NHPCO) reported that in 2018, 1.55 million Medicare beneficiaries received hospice care for an average of 3 months [23]. NHPCO also reported in a 2020 Palliative Care Needs Survey that almost 90,000 patients received palliative care services,

Table 1 Palliative and hospice resources	
Centers to Advance Palliative Care	Resources for providers: https://www.capc.org/
End-of-Life Nursing Education Consortium (ELNEC)	Resources for providers: https://www.aacnnursing.org/ELNEC
Get Palliative Care	Resources for patients and families: https://getpalliativecare.org
National Association of Areas on Aging	Resources for caregiver and transportation services: https://www.n4a.org/
National Hospice and Palliative Care Organization	Resources for providers and patients: https://www.nhpco.org/
National institute of nursing research	Resources for patient and caregiver education: https://www.ninr.nih.gov/newsandinformation/publications/palliative-care-resources

and that most of the care was provided by nurse practitioners [24]. Nurse practitioners should be familiar with community resources available for palliative care and hospice services. See Table 1 for a list of resources for providers, patients, and caregivers.

SUMMARY

Palliative care can be initiated at any stage of a chronic or life-limiting illness. Hospice care should be considered when a patient has an expected 6 months or less to live. Both palliative and hospice care can be provided in various settings. Before treatment begins, providers should thoroughly explain the expected disease trajectory to patients, the treatment and adverse effects, and whether the treatment can be expected to extend life. A goals of care discussion is indicated at diagnosis, as some patients are unwilling to disagree with the provider. In addition, patients often lack the knowledge to decipher whether a treatment will be too cumbersome or adversely affect his or her quality of life. Anxiety and depression are common in chronic illness states. While physical manifestations of illness are more easily detected and addressed, it is crucial for providers to regularly assess for anxiety and depression. The patient should be offered both pharmacologic and nonpharmacological treatment, such as counseling. Anxiety and depression in EOL care should be assessed and treated using a multidisciplinary approach.

CLINICS CARE POINTS

- All hospice care is palliative care; not all palliative care is hospice care.
- Palliative care can (and should) be initiated at the beginning of a life-limiting illness due to improved patient symptomatology and quality of life (QOL).

- Hospice care is reserved for patients with a life expectancy of less than 6 months.
- If a patient is admitted to hospice care and lives beyond the 6 month life expectancy, the patient is not automatically discharged. Following that time period, assessments are completed by a physician or nurse practitioner every 60 days to ensure the patient continues to meet criteria for services.

Disclosure

The author has no commercial or financial conflicts of interest or funding sources.

Reference List

[1] Depression and older adults. National Institute on Aging. Available at: https://www.nia.nih.gov/health/depression-and-older-adults. Accessed November 9, 2021.

[2] Kozlov E, Phongtankuel V, Prigerson H, et al. Prevalence, severity, and correlates of symptoms of anxiety and depression at the very end of life. J Pain Symptom Manage 2019;58(1): 80–5.

[3] van Oorschot B, Ishii K, Kusomoto Y, et al. Anxiety, depression and psychosocial needs are the most frequent concerns reported by patients: Preliminary results of a comparative explorative analysis of two hospital-based palliative care teams in Germany and Japan. J Neural Transm 2020;127(11):1481–9.

[4] Palliate definition and meaning. Dictionary.com. Available at: https://www.dictionary.com/browse/palliate. Accessed November 9, 2021.

[5] Palliative care for metastatic breast cancer. Breastcancer.org.. 2020. Available at: https://www.breastcancer.org/symptoms/types/recur_metast/stop_treat/palliative.   Accessed November 9, 2021.

[6] Shen MJ, Wellman JD. Evidence of palliative care stigma: the role of negative stereotypes in preventing willingness to use palliative care. Palliat Support Care 2019;17(04):374–80.

[7] Hawley P. Barriers to access to palliative care. Palliat Care Res Treat 2017;10:117822421668888.

[8] Hoerger M, Greer JA, Jackson VA, et al. Defining the elements of early palliative care that are associated with patient-reported outcomes and the delivery of end-of-life care. J Clin Oncol 2018;36(11):1096–102.

[9] Miller SC, Lima JC, Intrator O, et al. Palliative care consultations in nursing homes and reductions in acute care use and potentially burdensome end-of-life transitions. J Am Geriatr Soc 2016;64(11):2280–7.

[10] Sheridan PE, LeBrett WG, Triplett DP, et al. Cost savings associated with palliative care among older adults with advanced cancer. Am J Hosp Palliat Medicine 2021;38(10): 1250–7.

[11] Hospice. CMS. https://www.cms.gov/Medicare/Medicare-Fee-for-Service-Payment/Hospice. Accessed November 9, 2021.

[12] What are palliative care and hospice care? National Institute on Aging; 2021. https://www.nia.nih.gov/health/what-are-palliative-care-and-hospice-care. Accessed November 9, 2021.

[13] Levis B, Sun Y, He C, et al. Accuracy of the PHQ-2 alone and in combination with the PHQ-9 for screening to detect major depression. JAMA 2020;323(22):2290–300.

[14] Shin C, Park MH, Lee S-H, et al. Usefulness of the 15-item geriatric depression scale (gds-15) for classifying minor and major depressive disorders among community-dwelling elders. J Affect Disord 2019;259:370–5.

[15] Johnson SU, Ulvenes PG, Øktedalen T, et al. Psychometric properties of the General Anxiety Disorder 7-item (GAD-7) scale in a heterogeneous psychiatric sample. Front Psychol 2019;10:1713.

[16] Greer JA, Jacobs JM, El-Jawahri A, et al. Role of patient coping strategies in understanding the effects of early palliative care on quality of life and mood. J Clin Oncol 2018;36(1): 53–60.

[17] Rogers JG, Patel CB, Mentz RJ, et al. Palliative care in heart failure: the PAH-HF randomized, controlled trial. J Am Coll Cardiol 2017;70(3):331–41.

[18] Raj KS, Williams N, DeBattista C, et al. Psychiatric disorders. In: Papadakis MA, McPhee SJ, Rabow MW, editors. Current medical diagnosis & treatment 2021. New York: McGraw-Hill Education; 2021. p. 1082–137.

[19] Stahl SM, Pradko JF, Haight BR, et al. A review of the neuropharmacology of bupropion, a dual norepinephrine and dopamine reuptake inhibitor. The Prim Care Companion The J Clin Psychiatry 2004;06(04):159–66.

[20] Rabow MW, Pantilat SZ, Shah AC, et al. Palliative Care & Pain Management. In: Papadakis MA, McPhee SJ, Rabow MW, editors. Current medical diagnosis & treatment 2021. New York, (NY): McGraw-Hill Education; 2021. p. 70–101.

[21] Goldman N, Frankenthaler M, Klepacz L. The efficacy of ketamine in the palliative care setting: a comprehensive review of the literature. J Palliat Med 2019;22(9):1154–61.

[22] Wood H, Dickman A, Star A, et al. Updates in palliative care – overview and recent advancements in the pharmacological management of cancer pain. Clin Med 2018;18(1): 17–22.

[23] Hospice facts & figures. NHPCO. 2020. Available at: https://www.nhpco.org/factsfigures/. Accessed November 9, 2021.

[24] 2020 palliative care needs survey. NHPCO. 2020. Available at: https://www.nhpco.org/2020-pc-needs-survey/. Accessed November 9, 2021.

Culturally Informed Mental Health Care of Marginalized Older Adults

Tamatha Arms, PhD, DNP, PMHNP-BC, NP-C[a],*,
Linda J. Keilman, DNP, MSN, GNP-BC, FAANP[b],
George Byron Peraza-Smith, DNP, APRN-BC, GS-C, CNE,
FAANP[c]

[a]University of North Carolina Wilmington, CHHS School of Nursing, 601 South College Road, Wilmington, NC 28403, USA; [b]Michigan State University, College of Nursing, 1355 Bogue Street, A126 Life Science Building, East Lansing, MI 48824-1317, USA; [c]DNP & APRN Online Programs, South University, 709 Mall Bouvard, Savannah, GA 31406, USA

Keywords

• Culture • Culturally informed care • Marginalization • Mental health • Older adult
• Health care providers

Key points

• Culturally informed care is based on the recognition of facts that report specific groups and populations have historically had a marginalized status.

• Marginalization of older adults was apparent during the COVID-19 pandemic, partially through overt ageism and ableism.

• Culture is learned and constantly evolving.

• A minority group refers to individuals who share specific characteristics, including ethnicity.

• The advanced practice registered nurse has an obligation to be culturally aware, displaying cultural humility/respect, and value all components of cultural identity to provide quality culturally informed, culturally literate, care.

INTRODUCTION

Marginalization can be concerning related to cultural tendencies that associate shame and other negative consequences with seeking professional mental health assistance. Older adults (OA) may be included in marginalized groups related to physical limitation, socioeconomic status, cognitive issues, educational level,

*Corresponding author. E-mail address: armst@uncw.edu

https://doi.org/10.1016/j.yfpn.2021.12.002
2589-420X/22/© 2021 Elsevier Inc. All rights reserved.

culture, race, sexual identity/sexual preference, and specifically, mental health issues. Marginalized groups have been known as underserved, vulnerable, disregarded, persecuted, or sidelined, and they have existed for many years, especially related to immigrants, migrants, and refugees. Given that it would be impossible to include all potentially marginalized groups within this article, the focus is on the underserved OA groups of ethnic minorities, lesbian, gay, bisexual, transgender, and queer or questioning (LGBTQ)+ identified people, people who are homeless, and people who have an intellectual or developmental disorder.

MARGINALIZATION

To *marginalize* is a verb or an action "to relegate to an unimportant or powerless position within a society or group" [1]. To marginalize a group of people is to determine the group does not measure up to societal norms; therefore, the group is excluded from mainstream society [2]. *Marginalization* excludes some groups based on race, gender identity, sexual orientation, sexual preference, age, physical ability, cognitive status, mental health, language, religion, or immigration status [3]. Direct marginalization is explicit and obvious and regulates one to an unimportant or powerless position within a society or group. Indirect marginalization is implicit, with less obvious microaggressions. Marginalization can happen without mainstream society being aware of it [4]. Marginalization of OA before the COVID-19 pandemic focused on ageism, ableism, relativity or social exclusion, agency, dynamicity, and multidimensionality.

Domains of social exclusion include the following: (1) Neighborhood and community, (2) social relations, (3) services, (4) amenities and mobility, (5) material and financial resources, (6) sociocultural aspects, and (7) civic participation [5]. Since the COVID-19 pandemic, OA have faced further marginalization and mental health stigma. During the pandemic, it became widely known that OA were at greater risk for infection from the coronavirus; they were more likely to suffer higher mortalities and morbidities [6]. Some have coined this phenomenon the "gero-pandemic" [7]. Many societies have shunned those who are most susceptible to COVID-19, resulting in OA not seeking care at first signs or symptoms of COVID-19 because of fear of discriminatory behavior. OA have felt devalued, dehumanized, and rejected from family and society, as they have been isolated. This marginalization led to mental health issues of depression and anxiety, and in some cases, substance use disorders [7].

In this article, the focus is on marginalization of OA and mental health care. Mental health care should be considered in the context of each OA's unique characteristics, needs, individual preferences, ethnic background, culture, spiritual beliefs, and health literacy. These characteristics should be considered in support of *cultural respect* (CR), *cultural humility* (CH), dignity, autonomy, rights, equality, social justice, and unique individuality.

CULTURE

Culture is a dynamic multifactorial combination of beliefs, norms, values, ideas, customs, manners, habits, and behaviors passed on through generational written and spoken word over time. Culture is learned and constantly evolving. Although culture is unique to every individual, it involves specific elements from ethnic, racial, religious, geographic, or social groups [8]. An individual's culture can often be identified symbolically through language, behaviors, music, art, literature, food, clothing, jewelry, makeup, hair, mannerisms, and religion that is integrated into daily life. It is important to understand the characteristics of culture and how it is part of all human beings (Box 1).

Box 1: Characteristics of culture

- Learned
  - From families, peers, institutions, media
  - From enculturation: Process of learning/acquiring values and norms of the culture
  - Influences unconsciously [9]
- Adaptive
  - Taking on characteristics of a geographic region or country where one is living
  - Absorbing those characteristics of others that add value to one's primary culture
  - Gradually evolved and transformed over time
  - Never static for individuals or populations
- Shared
  - With other members of the population/community/group
  - Socially appropriate behavior that is predictable
  - Exposure to multiple cultures during a lifetime
- Based on symbols
  - Varied cross-culturally
  - Arbitrary
  - Patterns of behavior, actions, and so forth
  - Has meaning only when members agree on the use
  - Language is the most important symbol of culture
- Integrated and interrelated
  - Interconnected
  - Holistic
  - An interrelationship among all parts/components of culture
- Dynamic
  - Interactive, evolving
  - Exchange of ideas and symbols between groups [10]
  - Cultural processes and lived experiences that uniquely shape individuals [9]

Understanding how culture is learned and how integral it is to groups/populations leads to a deeper perspective on how culture impacts OA. One strategy to use with marginalized OA is to recognize their global view of life, health, and mental health, accomplished through CR and CH.

CR is recognizing inherent rights, values, traditions, and diversity of all unique individuals and is necessary to eradicate health disparities and provide quality care [8]. CR is taking the time to attentively listen, appropriately question, and explore all patients' needs, as the information contributes to the ability to meet diverse population and patient needs [11]. *CH* is committing to the lifelong pursuit of self-evaluation and ongoing critique of the inequities and disparities that impact people from specific populations and vowing to do something about the situation [12,13]. Tervalon and Murray-Garcia [11] believe CH is further understood to mean the development of mutually beneficial and nonpaternalistic partnerships with communities. CH also means adopting a personal practice philosophy that is other-oriented to aspects of cultural identity (CI) that are most important to the individual [12].

Openness as a health care provider (HCP) and incorporating the principles of CR and CH into one's practice philosophy will assist in understanding the health, healing, wellness, illness, disease, dying, and delivery of health services based on an individual's values and CI. CI is the self-conception and self-perception of feelings of belonging to a specific cultural or ethnic group [14]. Searching for self and belonging can be a lifelong process that is constantly changing based on explorations and discoveries of the individual on their quest. HCPs using culturally based engagement strategies with patients can have a positive impact on the establishment of therapeutic relationships and what the patient is willing to share [10–12,14]. CR enables health care systems, agencies, and HCP to understand and meet the needs of diverse populations seeking health information and care. The more HCP try to understand, the better HCP conversations will be understood and embraced by diverse patient populations. This phenomenon will lead to individualized treatment/management plans that are adhered to by patients because the plans incorporate cultural needs within the plan. Adhering to plans of care will lead to improved health outcomes and improved quality of life (QoL) for diverse patients [14]. Practicing from a person-centered model of CR and CH will lead to *culturally informed care* (CIC).

CIC is based on the following exemplars:

- Awareness of personal biases and beliefs
- Willingness
- Appreciation of otherness or being other-centered
- Use of inclusive language
- Fostering diversity
- Supporting social justice and equity [15]

CIC is also based on the recognition that specific groups and populations have historically had a marginalized status. Microaggressions and mistrust will impair a therapeutic alliance from forming and leave the person feeling disappointed, depressed, hopeless, having a lower self-esteem, having increased anxiety, and fearful of care [10].

There are multifactorial components of culture, including age, race, gender, education, religion, socioeconomic status, nationality, generation, ethnicity, sexual orientation, occupation, preferred language, spirituality, and advance care directives, to name a few. All are powerful influencers to every individual and their beliefs regarding health care. Table 1 lists and describes some of the principles/components of cultural domains [16–20].

CULTURE'S IMPACT ON HEALTH CARE

Does culture have an impact on mental health? Absolutely! Culture impacts health and health care through perceptions and meaning of health within a

Table 1	
Components or principles of culture	
Components/Principles	Meaning
• Race	• Narrow concept
	• Describes physical traits
	• Something you inherit
	• Based on similar physical & biological attributes [16]
• Ethnicity	• Broad concept
	• Based on cultural expression & place of origin
	• Cultural identification
	• Something you learn [16]
• Language	• Complex
	• Ingrained in culture
	• Linguistic competence
	• Art of communicating words, sounds, gestures; assumed by communities
	• Central to social life
	• Consider limited English proficiency [9]
• Religion, faith, spiritual beliefs	• Impact decisions related to nutrition, medication, modesty, preferred HCP gender [17]
	• important role in decision making
	• Provide guidance & emphasis on maintaining health
	• May impact attitudes & behaviors
	• Related to adherence & nonadherence of treatment plan
• Gender	• How one thinks about self & role (how "expected" to act, speak, dress, groom, & conduct self)
	• Gender identity (sex assignment) at birth
	• Culturally influenced stereotypes
	• Impacts decisions & behaviors
	• Expectations
	• Differentiation between femininity & masculinity
• Gender identity	• Internal concept of self
	• How one perceives themselves as male, female, a blend of both or neither
	• Can be same as sex assigned at birth or different [18]

(continued on next page)

Table 1
(continued)

Components/Principles	Meaning
• Gender expression	• External appearance of one's gender identity • Expressed through behavior, clothing, haircut, voice, & so forth • May or may not conform to socially defined behaviors & characteristics typically associated with being either masculine or feminine [18]
• Sexual orientation	• Inherent or immutable enduring emotional, romantic, or sexual attraction to other people [18]
• Socioeconomic status	• Strong determinant of lifespan health • Lower socioeconomic status associated with poorer health & greater psychological distress [19] • Related to support networks & access to material resources
• Age	• Length of time a person has been living • Based on birth date • With aging, there is decreased performance in cognitive domains, including speed of processing, working memory, long-term memory, reasoning
• Geographic origin	• Refers to region (place) of origin • Country in which the person comes from • Land, resource availability shape culture uniqueness
• Group history	• Several individuals assembled or having a unifying relationship [20]
• Education	• Process of gaining knowledge • Preservation of culture through instilling traditions, customs, values, arts, & so forth into learning • Transmit social values & ideals to members of society

cultural group. Culture will determine where, if, and from whom persons will seek care and their approach to health promotion and prevention [10]. Culture may define how illness, pain, mental disorders, and death are expressed and experienced as well as the causes of health and disease.

Culture gives significance to health information and messages. Perceptions and definitions of health and illness, preferences, language and cultural barriers, care process barriers, and stereotypes are all strongly influenced by culture and can have a great impact on health literacy and health outcomes [10,18]. Differing cultural and educational backgrounds among patients and providers, as well as among those who create health information and those who use it, contribute to problems with health literacy [20].

Culture provides a context through which meaning is gained from information and provides the purpose by which people come to understand their health status and comprehend options for diagnoses and treatments. A conceptual understanding of the interconnections between culture and literacy through the idea of *cultural literacy* can provide insights into the deeper meanings of how diverse populations in the United States come to know, comprehend, and make informed decisions based on valid data regarding their health [9,21].

Culture gives significance to health information and messages. Perceptions and definitions of health, illness and mental health, preferences, language and cultural barriers, care process barriers, and stereotypes are all strongly influenced by culture and can have a great impact on health literacy and health outcomes [21]. Differing cultural and educational backgrounds among patients and providers, as well as among those who create health information and those who use it, contribute to problems with health literacy. The relationship between culture, patient-provider interaction, and quality of care has been reviewed by Cooper and Roter [21]. Early work showed that European American cultural groups used language differently in discussing symptoms, such as pain [22,23]. These linguistic differences were associated with differences in diagnoses, irrespective of symptoms. African American (AA) patients frequently experience shorter physician-patient interactions and less patient-centered visits than Caucasian patients [9,22,24,25].

Mental health disorders are more prevalent in minority OA populations, especially AA [26]. A *minority* is a segment of the overall population that is different from others based on specific characteristics and are often treated differently than the majority, or in other words, marginalized [27]. A *minority group* refers to individuals who share characteristics, such as race, ethnicity, culture, values, religion, disability, gender, sexual orientation, socioeconomic status, and health. In 1958, Wagley and Harris [27] determined the following 5 characteristics that define a minority group:

1. Distinguishing physical or cultural traits (ie, skin color, language)
2. Unequal treatment and less power over their lives
3. Involuntary membership in the group
4. Awareness of subordination
5. High rate of in-group marriage [28,29]

OA are considered a minority group. Culture, race, and ethnicity affect aging. Racial and ethnic-minority OA are the fastest growing population in the United States, especially those over the age of 85 [26]. As this population increases, it is a demographic imperative that HCP understand more about who these OA are to provide individualized, person-centered, values-driven, culturally competent, quality care. Nurse practitioners need to understand the *culture of prejudice* (CoP) that exists in the US health care system [11,26,29]. CoP refers to the theory that prejudice is embedded in US culture [30]. Growing up in the United States exposes many to stereotypes, casual racial imagery, and myths about minority groups [29,30]. How does this exposure influence the way prejudice or bias becomes a part of HCP thought processes? More research is needed in this area. However, what we do know is that psychopathology leading to mental health disorders is impacted by race, ethnic, and cultural factors [26,28]. In addition, there are historical, intergenerational, and social challenges that stem from social determinants of health (SDOH).

SOCIAL DETERMINATES OF HEALTH

According to the US Department of Health and Human Services and Healthy People 2030, "SDOH are the conditions in the environments where people are born, live, learn, work, play, worship, and age that affect a wide range of health, functioning, and QoL outcomes and risks" [31]. The 5 domains of SDOH are as follows:

- Economic stability
- Education access and quality
- Health care access and quality
- Neighborhood and built environment
- Social and community context [31]

In addition to SDOH, there are social determinants of mental health (SDoMH) that encompass the social and socioeconomic domains that adversely impact mental health disparities [32].

Mental health is defined as a person's overall well-being and the ability to maintain activities of daily living and instrumental activities of daily living [32]. Mental health is guided by biological, environmental, and socioeconomic factors [32]. Perhaps it is most important for HCP to know that poor mental health is associated with rapid social change, stressful work conditions or no work, gender discrimination, ageism, social exclusion or isolation, unhealthy lifestyle, physical ill health, and violations of human rights [33]. Given all of the social determinants, it is imperative to know the person's story in order to know the individual and garner from them their life goals, values, and wishes for their health. SDOH are well documented regarding the conditions over which the individual has little or no control but that affect his or her ability to participate fully in a health-literate society [9].

Consider Fig. 1. What constructs do you think need to be added?

The term *intersectionality* is not without controversy. Coined in 1989 when written in an academic paper [34], the word has transformed in the last 3 decades to basically mean every individual has a unique identity that intersects in a variety of ways that impact how the individual is viewed, understood, and treated. The hope of understanding this concept is to become aware of this phenomenon and advocate and empower others to create a leveled playing field for equity and social justice in health care, politics, law, and living every day. Related to this article, SDOH and SDoMH intersect in all ways; the head and heart are not separate from the body and the environment in which all individuals live, grow, and die. Understanding the individual OA story is to understand their life-long journey related to SDOH and SDoMH and to determine how best to diagnose, treat, and manage any mental health issues they may live with.

MENTAL HEALTH AND OLDER ADULTS

Positive mental health has a significant effect on achieving a positive sense of well-being. Mental health and physical health have a synergistic effect on aging.

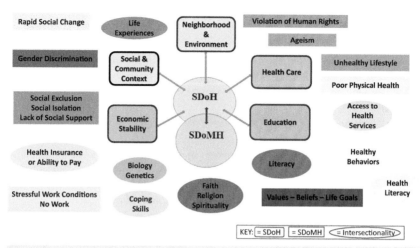

Fig. 1. SDoH and SDoMH intersectionality.

This synergistic effect can be either a positive or a negative experience. Mental health and mental illness are stigmatized by society, leading to a compounding destructive impact of mental health with aging. Add to this mix, an OA and mental health who is in a marginalized group, and the effect can be devastating, leading to being isolated and ostracized. This triple compounding effect prevents many OA belonging to marginalized groups from trusting and seeking medical help, especially for mental health conditions.

According to the Gerontological Advanced Practice Nursing Association Geropsychiatric Nursing Position Statement, primary care providers serve as gatekeepers and provide access to mental health care for OA [35]. Providers have a professional obligation to examine their unique individual prejudices and preconceived notions of the intersection between aging, mental health, and marginalized groups. HCPs and practice settings need to create environments that are welcoming to all by identifying and removing barriers. Marginalized OA are sensitive to the signs that a practice is open and inclusive to them (Box 2).

Discrimination, stereotypes, and prejudice toward OA are a result of a society that values youth over aging. The devaluing of aging has created barriers to inclusive, quality health care resulting in health inequalities, disparities, and negative impacts on outcomes for OA [36]. *Ageism* in the context of this article is the negative impact of stereotypes and prejudices held by persons based on the chronologic age of an individual [37]. Adding mental health conditions to the negative impact of ageism is associated with preventing or delaying health care access [38].

Risk factors to consider for mental health with marginalized groups are listed in Box 3.

Box 2: Questions practice settings need to address when creating inclusive environments for marginalized older adults

- Are there clearly posted, visible, and in large print nondiscrimination statements on the walls and in patient rooms?
- Are the waiting and reception areas open to a variety of individuals and backgrounds?
- Do intake forms acknowledge an inclusive acceptance of representative groups and lifestyles?
- Are there visual cues in displays, posters, and brochures that cover the health concerns of various groups? Do patients and families see themselves represented?
- Does the practice include symbols and representation of all groups?
- Are the providers and staff from admission through discharge aware and respectful of different groups?
- Do the providers and staff reflect and represent the groups they are treating?
- Are providers and staff aware of personal biases and attitudes toward a marginalized group?
- Are providers and staff actively working to prevent these biases from impacting interactions, treatments, and health outcomes?
- Does the practice follow best practices in hiring the appropriate providers and staff with shared values?
- Have the providers and staff received education/training on effective communication and management of various marginalized groups, including ageism?

OLDER ADULT IMMIGRANTS/MINORITIES

Segregating care and managing a group of OA based on stereotyped ideals lead to marginalization. Marginalized OA are heterogeneous groups with unique physical and mental health issues that require recognition to optimize medical and mental health assessment and culturally sensitive treatment [39]. The

Box 3: Risk factors for mental health

- Medical comorbidities
- Loss of independence
- Loss of close friends or family members
- Decrease in economic status
- Loneliness or social isolation
- Extended periods of heightened stress
- Elder abuse or neglect
- Poor nutrition
- Significant family history and exposure

consideration for potential biases when conducting a geriatric comprehensive assessment is an important step toward providing appropriate, person-centered, and antioppressive care. HCPs must commit to nondiscriminatory, antioppressive practices when addressing issues of ethnicity and culture as part of mental health assessment and treatment of marginalized OA. Immigrants who are OA experience stigma and limited access to mental health services. OA immigrants are challenged with understanding the cultural norms differently from their own while attempting to navigate through a complex health care system. This barrier is intensified when attempting to access and use mental health services.

There are unique challenges for immigrant OA, including lack of insurance, lack of access, cost of mental health treatments, and language barriers [40]. The HCP may need to take more time and use a professional interpreter. The HCP should discover the cultural implications of mental health within the immigrant's home country and culture. It is critical to connect the immigrant OA with comprehensive community-based and health care services. The HCP should become knowledgeable regarding immigrant cultures and be sensitive to their needs. Some immigrants will seek traditional healers and may desire to integrate the healers and providers treatment. Awareness and sensitivity are key.

OLDER VETERANS

US service veterans are not often seen as a marginalized group. However, military veterans receiving mental health services in the community often feel marginalized. Many veterans returning from service may feel isolated, finding the transition from service back to their community challenging. Veterans report the transition to civilian life can be difficult with establishing or reestablishing friendships, reconnecting with family, and being isolated from the community [41] Although service members share a common culture, their individual experiences can vary tremendously depending on the military branch served, length and location of service, and the level of combat interface. Many OA veterans with mental health issues may experience compounding overlapping vulnerabilities related to race/ethnic and sexual minorities. Almost half of the US veterans are older than 65 years of age; they are at higher risk for mental health conditions, which are associated with increased mortality and health care costs [42].

Older veterans with posttraumatic stress disorders and other mental health issues are the most likely to be isolated and experience more interpersonal relationship problems [43]. Many older veterans have benefited from the shared experience and reflection of the wartime experience with fellow older veterans, which provided mechanisms for coping and placing the wartime experience into perspective. However, as the older veteran ages, there are fewer shared connections, as the older veteran is more connected to their communities and less to Veterans Administration (VA) services. This loss of connection and shared experiences further serves to isolate the older veteran. Older veterans receiving mental services in the community are significantly lower and have significantly higher dropout rates than the general public [44]. A major barrier to older veterans seeking mental health treatment is related to stigma [45,46]. HCPs who work with older veterans must be cognizant of their unique needs for mental health services (Box 4). Many veterans use an HPC in the community. A useful VA tool kit resource for community primary care providers can be found at https://www.mentalhealth.va.gov/communityproviders/

OLDER LESBIAN, GAY, BISEXUAL, TRANSGENDER, AND QUEER OR QUESTIONING + INDIVIDUALS

There are no reliable demographic data sets on the actual number of sexual minorities in the United States, and even fewer pieces of data on OA who are LGBTQ+. Most projections are that 4% to 10% of the population are LGBTQ+ [47]. The definitions for sexual minorities have changed considerably over the past few decades, and newer generations view sexuality as a more fluid construct than previous generations. However, the LGBTQ+ OA have been oppressed and discriminated against for their sexual orientation for decades, and perhaps a lifetime. LGBTQ + OA lived through during a time when being an identified LGBTQ + person meant being ostracized, seen as defected, and immoral. Many state laws prohibited acts of homosexuality. This older generation of LGBTQ + experienced a higher level of margination than the current generation.

Box 4: Questions practice settings need to consider when creating inclusive environments for older veterans with mental health conditions

- Do you know the cultures and subcultures as well as the mission and core values of the branch of military services of your patients?
- Are the providers and staff familiar with the culture and language specific to military veterans?
- Do intake forms acknowledge an inclusive acceptance of the veteran and service branch?
- Is there space for addressing the potential of moral injury related to service addressed in the care of the veteran?
- Are providers respectful of the veteran and seek permission to ask about their military service? Does the intake include military service history?
- Does the veteran's military service have an impact on their health care engagement and behaviors (Warrior Ethos)?
- Is the practice aware and connected to veteran-centric resources?
- Are staff knowledgeable about the types of veteran-centric services available to older veterans?

Adapted from Richard-Eaglin A, Campbell JG, Utley-Smith Q. The aging veteran population: Promoting awareness to influence best practices. Geriatr Nurs. 2020;41(4);505-507. https://www.sciencedirect.com/science/article/abs/pii/S0197457220301920; with permission

Marginalized OA identifying as LGBTQ + represent a diverse spectrum of individuals and groups. The OA who identifies as LGBTQ + has unique health care needs. LGBTQ + OA have 2 to 3 times higher incidences of depression, anxiety, and suicidal ideation than the majority public [47]. LGBTQ + OA may not be as open about their sexuality with providers and staff because of fear of being rejected and receiving subpar health care. HCP can create a welcoming environment for LGBTQ + OA and promote a safe harbor for receiving health care. First, all HCPs and staff must examine their own biases and homophobia/heterosexism. Demonstrating acceptance of the LGBTQ + OA, while being sensitive to their privacy needs, can help create a trusting relationship.

CLINICAL PRACTICE IMPLICATIONS

Marginalization manifestation is as follows:

- Ageist
- Use of derogatory language
- Stereotypes
- Judging identity
- Inequity access related to resources (barriers to access and support)
- Assuming preferred pronouns and/or sexual orientation/preference
- Not understanding, caring, or being aware of a person's cultural or religious traditions and values [48–50]

Manifestations result in anger, apathy, anxiety, fear, depression, mistrust, paranoia, psychosis, hopelessness, powerlessness, spiritual distress, and social isolation. Unfortunately, OA are marginalized in various groups in society. Some are in multiple marginalized groups. Being marginalized impacts mental health and resilience. Culture makes a difference in all marginalized groups. HCPs should be educated to provide CIC to all individuals, including patients. HCPs who are not competent to provide CIC should place appropriate referrals for the OA's best interest.

SUMMARY

In this article, the authors tried to present foundational information important to providing quality, holistic, person-centered, CIC. Although the focus was on the marginalization of OA, the concepts of CH, CI, cultural literacy, and CR intersect the lives of all individuals across the lifespan. To move forward, take time to evaluate your knowledge, values, and feelings about culture, marginalization, and the US health care system. What can you do to make the system better? What are you already doing to make a positive impact? How can you create an even stronger bond with your patients in helping them to gain optimal health? How will you take the information from this article and move the US health care system forward? YOU can make a difference!

CLINICS CARE POINTS

- Cultural respect varies from cultural humility, culturally informed care, and cultural literacy.
- The goal of every practitioner should be to practice culturally informed care.
- Box 2 provides a list of evidence-based activities a clinical practice can do to create inclusive environments for marginalized older adults.

References

[1] Merriam-Webster. Marginalize. Available at: https://www.merriam-webster.com/dictionary/marginalize. Accessed September 7, 2021.

[2] Abbott P, Sapsford R. Marginalization. Encyclopedia of gerontology and population aging 2019. Available at: https://link.springer.com/referenceworkentry/10.1007%2F978-3-319-69892-2_501-1 Accessed August 1, 2020.

[3] Sevelius JM, Gutierrez-Mock L, Zamuiod-Haas S, et al. Research with marginalized communities: challenges to continuity during the COVID-19 pandemic. AIDS Behav 2020;5(16):1–4. Available at: https://link.springer.com/article/10.1007/s10461-020-02920-3.

[4] Hartblay C. After marginalization: pixelization, disability, and social difference in digital Russia. SAQ 2019;118(3):543–72. Available at: https://www.academia.edu/40095192/After_Marginalization_Pixelization_Disability_and_Social_Difference_in_Digital_Russia.

[5] D'Cruz M, Banerjee D. 'An invisible human rights crisis': the marginalization of older adults during the COVID-19 pandemic – an advocacy review. Psychiatry Res 2020;292:113369. Available at: https://www.meta.org/papers/an-invisible-human-rights-crisis-the/32795754.

[6] Tehrani H. Mental health stigma related to novel coronavirus disease (COVID-19) in older adults. Geriatr Gerontol Int 2020;20(8):796–7. Available at: https://www.ncbi.nlm.nih.gov/pmc/articles/PMC7361788/.

[7] Wister A, Speechley M. COVID-19: pandemic risk, resilience and possibilities for aging research. Can J Aging 2020;39(3):344–7. Available at: https://pubmed.ncbi.nlm.nih.gov/32423497/.

[8] National Institutes of Health. Cultural respect. 2021. Available at: https://www.nih.gov/institutes-nih/nih-office-director/office-communications-public-liaison/clear-communication/cultural-respect. Accessed September 7, 2021.

[9] Nielsen-Bohlman L, Panzer AM, Kindig DA, editors. Health literacy: a prescription to end confusion. Washington, DC: Institute of Medicine Committee on Health Literacy of the National Academies; 2004. Available at: https://pubmed.ncbi.nlm.nih.gov/25009856/. Accessed September 7, 2021.

[10] Nideffer RF. The characteristics of culture. Available at: https://nideffer.net/classes/GCT_RPI_S14/readings/Chap8CharacteristicsofCulture.htm. Accessed September 6, 2021.

[11] Tervalon M, Murray-Garcia J. Cultural humility versus cultural competence: a critical distinction in defining physician training outcomes in multicultural education. J Health Care Poor Underserved 1998;9(2):117–25. Available at: https://muse.jhu.edu/article/268076/-summary?casa_token=Dobj81-vf-EAAAAA:kNcX1USpn59a6cA_93R784jVAJy8wb0HparE_K0AtoNrlmOm__hTgin10Fm1STq7gsfdKMzl0w.

[12] Hook JN, Davis DE, Owen J, et al. Cultural humility: measuring openness to culturally diverse clients. J Couns Psychol 2013;60(3):353–66. Available at: https://psycnet.apa.org/doiLanding?doi=10.1037%2Fa0032595.

[13] White AA, Logghe HJ, Goodenough DA, et al. Self-awareness and cultural identity as an effort to reduce bias in medicine. J Racial Ethn Health Disparities 2018;5:34–49. Available at: https://pubmed.ncbi.nlm.nih.gov/28342029/. Accessed September 6, 2021.

[14] Tadros E, Owens D. Clinical implications for culturally informed counseling with incarcerated individuals. Am J Fam Ther 2020;49(4):344–5. Available at: https://www.tandfonline.com/doi/full/10.1080/01926187.2020.1813659?casa_token=F87yRLZDAwAAAAA%3AAmUG_76GpbA1cN5I9J5IBTrmkD2fDbW0pRWgMKWdHP_PzBkdyeyy7LXQTFJOc-bmsjuSgSL7ClOR. Accessed June 20, 2021.

[15] Morin A. The difference between race and ethnicity. Verywellmind.com. 2020. Available at: https://www.verywellmind.com/difference-between-race-and-ethnicity-5074205. Accessed June 20, 2021.

[16] Swihart DL, Yarrarapu SNS, Martin RL. Cultural religious competence in clinical practice. Treasure Island, Florida: StatPearls Publishing; 2018. Available at: https://europepmc.org/article/NBK/nbk493216. Accessed June 26, 2021.

[17] Human Rights Campaign. Sexual orientation and gender identity definitions. n.d. Available at: https://www.hrc.org/resources/sexual-orientation-and-gender-identity-terminology-and-definitions. Accessed August 29, 2021.

[18] Milas G, Martinovic Klaric I, Malnar A, et al. Socioeconomic status, social-cultural values, life stress, and health behaviors in a national sample of adolescents. Stress Health 2019;35(2):217–24. Available at: https://pubmed.ncbi.nlm.nih.gov/30609225/.

[19] Merriam-Webster Dictionary. Group. Available at: https://www.merriam-webster.com/dictionary/group. Accessed August 29, 2021.

[20] Scrimshaw SC. Science, health, and cultural literacy in a rapidly changing communications landscape. PNAS 2019;116(16):7650–5. Available at: https://www.pnas.org/content/116/16/7650. Accessed September 7, 2021.

[21] Cooper LA, Roter DL. Patient-provider communication: the effect of race and ethnicity on process and outcomes of healthcareInstitute of Medicine (US) Committee on Understanding and Eliminating Racial and Ethnic Disparities in Health Care. In: Smedley BD, Stith AY, Nelson AR, editors. Unequal treatment: confronting racial and ethnic disparities in health care. Washington, DC: Institute of Medicine, The National Academies Press; 2003. Available at: https://www.ncbi.nlm.nih.gov/books/NBK220354/.

[22] Zborowski M. Cultural components in responses to pain. J Social Issues 1952;8(4):16–30. Available at: https://spssi.onlinelibrary.wiley.com/doi/10.1111/j.1540-4560.1952.tb01860.x.

[23] Zola IK. Culture and symptoms-an analysis of patient's presenting complaints. Am Sociol Rev 1966;31:615–30. Available at: https://psycnet.apa.org/record/1967-01861-001.

[24] Cooper-Patrick L, Gallo JJ, Gonzales JJ, et al. Race, gender, and partnership in the patient-physician relationship. JAMA 1999;282(6):583–9. Available at: https://jamanetwork.com/journals/jama/fullarticle/191132.

[25] Trinh NT, Bernard-Negron R, Ahmed I. Mental health issues in racial and ethnic minority elderly. Curr Psychiatry Rep 2019;21:100–6. Available at: https://pubmed.ncbi.nlm.nih.gov/31522260/.

[26] Merriam Webster. (n.d.). Minority. Available at: https://www.merriam-webster.com/dictionary/minority Accesed August 1, 2020.

[27] Wagley C, Harris M. Minorities in the new world: six case studies. New York: Columbia University Press; 1964.

[28] Northern Essex Community CollegeAsha Lal Tamang, Minneapolis Community and Technical College & North Hennepin Community College Contributing Authors Jennifer Hensley, Vincennes University Jennifer L. Trost, University of St. ThomasPamela Alcasey, Central Texas CollegeKate McGonigal, Fort Hays State University Heather Griffiths, Fayetteville State University Nathan Keirns, Zane State CollegeEric Strayer, Hartnell CollegeTommy Sadler, Union UniversitySusan Cody-Rydzewski, Georgia Perimeter CollegeGail Scaramuzzo, Lackawanna CollegeSally Vyain, Ivy Tech Community CollegeJeff Bry, Minnesota

State Community and Technical College at MoorheadFaye Jones, Mississippi Gulf Coast Community College. In: Conerly TR, Holmes K, Tamang AL, editors. Introduction to sociology. 3rd edition. Houston (TX): OpenStax; 2021. p. 289–328.

[29] Sorenson JS. Either you are with us or you are the terrorists. In: Blackwell JC, Smith M, editors. Culture of prejudice: arguments in critical social science. 2nd edition. Toronto (Canada): University of Toronto Press; 2003. p. 67–73. Available at: https://www.jstor.org/stable/10.3138/j.ctt2ttwcm.

[30] U.S. Department of Health and Human Services, Office of Disease Prevention and Health Promotion. Healthy People 2030: social determinants of health. Available at: https://health.gov/healthypeople/objectives-and-data/social-determinants-health. Accessed October 30, August 29, 2010.

[31] Fink-Samnick E. The social determinants of mental health: definitions, distinctions, and dimensions for professional case management: part 1. Prof Case Manage 2021;25(3): 121–37.

[32] World Health Organization. Mental health: strengthening our response. 2018. Available at: https://www.who.int/news-room/fact-sheets/detail/mental-health-strengthening-our-response. Accessed October 30, 2021.

[33] Crenshaw K. She coined the term 'intersectionality' over 30 years ago: here's what it means to her today. Time, Inc.; 2021. Available at: https://time.com/5786710/kimberle-crenshaw-intersectionality/.

[34] Gerontological Advanced Practice Nurses Association. GAPNA geropsychiatric nursing position statement: supporting evidence for geropsychiatric nursing as a subspeciality of gerontological advanced practice nursing. Reviewed June 21, 2021. 2019. Available at: https://www.gapna.org. Accessed October 30, 2021.

[35] Chang ES, Kannoth S, Levy S, et al. Global reach of ageism on older persons' health: a systemic review. PLoS ONE 2020;15(1):e0220857. Available at: https://journals.plos.org/plosone/article?id=10.1371/journal.pone.0220857.

[36] Mehri S, Hosseini MA, Shahbelaghi FM, et al. Explaining nurses' perception of the causes of ageism in hospital settings. Electron J Gen Med 2020;17(5):em218. Available at: https://www.ejgm.co.uk/article/explaining-nurses-perception-of-the-causes-of-ageism-in-hospital-settings-7881. Accessed August 27, 2021.

[37] Temple JB, Brijnath B, Enticott J, et al. Discrimination reported by older adults living with mental health conditions: Types, context, and association with healthcare barriers. Soc Psychiatry Psychiatr Epidemiol 2021;56:1003–14. Available at: https://pubmed.ncbi.nlm.nih.gov/32696302/. Accessed August 27, 2021.

[38] Veltman A, La Rose T. Marginalized geriatric patients. In: Hategan A, Bourgeois J, Hirsch C, et al, editors. Int. J. Geriatr. Psychiatry. Springer; 2018. p. 2021. Available at: https://link.springer.com/chapter/10.1007/978-3-319-67555-8_30. Accessed August 27, 2021.

[39] Fendian C. Mental healthcare for immigrants and first-generation families: erasing the stigma and creating solutions. J Health Care L Policy 2021;24:1–25. Available at: https://digitalcommons.law.umaryland.edu/cgi/viewcontent.cgi?article=1399&context=jhclp.

[40] Mamon D, Scoglio AAJ, Calixte RM, et al. Connecting veterans and their community through narrative: pilot data on a community strengthening intervention. Community Ment Health J 2020;56:804–13. Available at: https://pubmed.ncbi.nlm.nih.gov/31907805/.

[41] Atkinson DM, Donane BM, Thuras PD, et al. Mental health diagnoses in veterans referred to outpatient geriatric psychiatric care at a Veteran Affairs medical center. Mil Med 2020;185(3/4):e347. Available at: https://academic.oup.com/milmed/article/185/3-4/e347/5588771.

[42] Goldberg J, Magruder KM, Forsberg CW, et al. Prevalence of posttraumatic stress disorder in aging Vietnam-era veterans: Veterans Administration Cooperative Study 569: course and consequences of posttraumatic stress disorder in Vietnam-era veteran twins. Am J Geriatr Psychiatry 2014;24:181–91. Available at: https://pubmed.ncbi.nlm.nih.gov/26560508/.

[43] Cully JA, Tolpin L, Henderson L, et al. Psychotherapy in the Veterans Health Administration: missed opportunities? Psychol Serv 2018;5:320–31. Available at: https://www.ncbi.nlm.nih.gov/pmc/articles/PMC4145407/.

[44] Johnson EM, Possemato K. Problem recognition and treatment beliefs relate to mental health utilization among veteran primary care patients. Psychol Serv 2021;18(1):11–22. Available at: https://pubmed.ncbi.nlm.nih.gov/30869974/.

[45] Richard-Eaglin A, Campbell JG, Utley-Smith Q. The aging veteran population: promoting awareness to influence best practices. Geriatr Nurs 2020;41(4):505–7. Available at: https://www.sciencedirect.com/science/article/abs/pii/S0197457220301920.

[46] King M, Semlyen J, See Tai S, et al. Mental disorders, suicide, and deliberate self-harm in lesbian, gay and bisexual people: a systematic review of the literature. 2009. Department of Mental Health Sciences, Royal Free and University College Medical School, University College London. Available at: https://bmcpsychiatry.biomedcentral.com/articles/10.1186/1471-244X-8-70 Accesed October 1, 2020.

[47] Le Cook B, Trinh N, Li Z, et al. Trends in racial-ethnic disparities in access to mental health care, 2004-2012. Psychiatr Serv 2016;68(1). Available at: https://ps.psychiatryonline.org/doi/full/10.1176/appi.ps.201500453. Accessed September 1, 2021.

[48] Cuellar NG. Marginalization of cultural groups. J Transcult Nurs 2016;27(2):93. Available at: https://journals.sagepub.com/doi/full/10.1177/1043659615627495.

[49] Knaak S, Mantler E, Szeto A. Mental illness-related stigma in healthcare: barriers to access and care and evidence-based solutions. Healthc Manage Forum 2017;30(2):111–6. Available at: https://journals.sagepub.com/doi/full/10.1177/0840470416679413.

[50] Centers for Disease Control and Prevention. Basics of COVID-19. Updated May 24, 2021. Available at: https://www.cdc.gov/coronavirus/2019-ncov/your-health/about-covid-19/basics-covid-19.html. Accessed October 30, 2021.

The Medicare Wellness Visit
A Time to Address Mental Health and Well-Being

Rhonda Wells Lucas, MSN, AGPCNP-BC, GS-C[a],*,
Janice Taylor, DNP, AGPCNP-BC[b],
Laurie Kennedy-Malone, PhD, GNP-BC[c,d]

[a]Optum HouseCalls, 6675 Business Parkway Suite F, Elkridge, MD 21075, USA; [b]UAMS College of Nursing, 4301 West Markham Street Slot #529, Little Rock, AR 72205, USA; [c]UNCG School of Nursing, Nursing and Instructional Building, 1007 Walker Avenue, Greensboro, NC 27412, USA; [d]UNCG School of Nursing, PO Box 26170, Greensboro, NC 27402-6170, USA

Keywords

• Medicare Annual Wellness Visit • Screening • Mental health

Key points

• Reviewing the older adult's risk assessment for mental health disorders is a required component of the Medicare Annual Wellness Visit.
• Depression is a required screening of the Medicare Annual Wellness Visit.
• Positive findings identified as part of the mental health screenings trigger further exploration of the social determinants of health on the patient's well-being.

INTRODUCTION

Although it has been more than 50 years since the bill that enacted Medicare (MC) in the United States was signed into law in 1965, it was not until the last 10 years that a provision was established that provides a mechanism for structured comprehensive screening geared toward prevention. Every MC recipient is provided the opportunity to participate in the Annual Wellness Visit (AWV) by a licensed provider, that is, physician, nurse practitioner (NP), clinical nurse specialist, or physician assistant. The addition of the AWV as a benefit of all MC recipients was included in The Patient Protection

The authors do not have any financial relationships to disclose.

*Corresponding author. E-mail address: jewels4encouragement@gmail.com

and Affordable Care Act, along with the Health Care and Education Reconciliation Act of 2010 amendment, signed into law by President Barack Obama [1].

The AWV includes preventative screening by the person's provider and/or insurance company provider both initially and then annually. If the visit is conducted by the provider in a clinic or office, it is available after the recipient has MC Part B greater than 12 months. This annual visit is free to the MC client without deductible and is a billable visit by the provider. The AWV is not to be confused with the Welcome to MC Visit, also called the Initial Preventive Physical Examination, which includes a head-to-toe examination and is completed within the first 12 months of MC coverage [1]. Most of the major MC Complete insurance providers either contract with or hire NP, PA, and/ or physicians to conduct these visits in the MC recipient's home. The benefit may be available as soon as the recipient's MC Part B is effective.

The AWV is an overview of the patient's health, focusing on the development of a plan to keep the individual healthy. The visit includes assessments of the older adult's health; psychosocial risks and behavioral risks; cognitive and physical functioning; and ability to perform activities of daily living (ADL), fall risk, body mass index (BMI), and vital signs. At the conclusion of the visit, the provider and the MC recipient, together, formulate a plan for preventative health screenings, lifestyle interventions, and goals for wellness [2]. The AWV screening targets areas that may not normally in the past have been screened for in annual examination in primary care, namely depression [3]. A comprehensive screening approach toward understanding a patient's mental health and well-being is now required to be completed at the AWV for all MC recipients [2,4]. (Box 1).

SCREENING FOR MENTAL HEALTH ISSUES DURING THE ANNUAL WELLNESS VISIT: CASE PERSPECTIVES

Medicare complete nurse practitioner Annual Wellness Visit: value of home visit

Mrs G is an obese 80-year-old White widow who lives in a duplex in rural North Carolina. Mrs G is a new patient whose MC Complete insurance company arranges for the AWV to be conducted in the participant's home over the span of approximately 60 minutes. On arrival to Mrs G's home, the NP verified her identity. She meets the NP at the door smiling and invites the provider into her home.

Fall and functional assessments

As the visit begins, the NP questions the patient about the past 12 months, and Mrs G reveals that she had recently fallen and was still experiencing left knee pain. She explained further that it was difficult for her to get around since the fall. It was noted she moves slowly holding on to furniture for support. Mrs G stated that a year ago, she was getting around well and was "strong." Falls can be common in the older adult and contribute to increased mortality, morbidity, and use of medical services in this age group [2]. A fall risk assessment

Box 1: Components of the Annual Wellness Visit that address mental health and well-being

A review of any current opioid prescriptions means, with respect to the individual determined to have a current prescription for opioids, all of the following:

- A review of the potential risk factors to the individual for opioid use disorder
- An evaluation of the individual's severity of pain current treatment plan
- The provision of information on nonopioid treatment options
- A referral to a pain specialist, as appropriate

Detection of any cognitive impairment obtained by way of patient report and concerns raised by family members, friends, caretakers, or others.

- Review (administration if needed) of a health risk assessment
- Detection of any cognitive impairment
- Review of the individual's potential risk factors for depression, including current or past experiences with depression or other mood disorders, based on the use of an appropriate screening instrument for persons without a current diagnosis of depression
- Age-appropriate preventive services covered by MC
- A list of risk factors conditions for which primary, secondary, or tertiary interventions are recommended or are underway for the individual, including any mental health conditions or any such risk factors or conditions that have been identified through an initial preventive physical examination
- Reducing identified risk factors improving self-management or community-based lifestyle interventions to reduce health risks promote self-management wellness, including weight loss, physical activity, smoking cessation, fall prevention, and nutrition. Furnishing of a review of any current opioid prescriptions as that term is defined in this section
- Screening for potential substance use disorders including a review of the individual's potential risk factors for substance use disorder referral for treatment as appropriate
- Self-assessment of health status, frailty, and physical functioning
- Psychosocial risks, including but not limited to, depression/life satisfaction, stress, anger, loneliness/social isolation, pain, and fatigue
- Behavioral risks, including but not limited to, tobacco use, physical activity, nutrition oral health, alcohol consumption, sexual health, motor vehicle safety (seat belt use), and home safety
- Any other element determined appropriate through the national coverage determination process

Adapted from Medicare Wellness Visits. https://www.cms.gov/Outreach-and-Education/Medicare-Learning-Network-MLN/MLNProducts/preventive-services/medicare-wellness-visits.html. Accessed November 23, 2021; with permission.

developed by the insurance company by whom the NP was used was completed. The assessment inquired about the number of falls in the last 12 months, presence of any foot numbness, use of any durable medical equipment (ie, walker or cane), and any feeling of unsteadiness while walking. Mrs G scored yes on all except for foot numbness, flagging her as high risk for falls. She did state her primary care provider (PCP) was aware she is at fall risk and that she uses her cane and "was as careful as I could be" following fall precautions. She was asked about treatment of the knee, and she informed the NP she was seeing an orthopedic surgeon, getting joint injections every 3 to 4 months, and wearing a brace for a torn left meniscus. Many falls do not cause injuries, but when an older adult suffers injuries as a result of a fall, it makes it hard for a person to be mobile and independent in instrumental ADL (IADL).

Pain assessment
In assessing pain, Mrs G stated she had achy pain on both sides of her left knee that, at times, would "shoot" across her knee and down her leg. She rated her pain 7 at the time of the visit, with it being a 4 at best and 10 at its worst. Mrs G stated her pain was "tolerable" taking 2 extra strength acetaminophen (650 mg tablets) twice daily for the last 6 months. She also stated that the knee injections by the orthopedic surgeon were helpful in controlling her pain but were "not lasting as long now" with the return of pain within 6 weeks or so.

Medication review
A medication reconciliation indicated Mrs G was taking alprazolam for anxiety and had been on this medication for "at least 30 years." The NP reviewed with her about how anxiolytics can cause imbalance, which may result in unsteadiness that could increase her chance for falls [2]. Mrs G agreed to speak with her PCP about weaning off the alprazolam that she takes at night to help her sleep. Mrs G was on several blood pressure medications and metformin but denied dizziness or hypoglycemic episodes.

History and preventative screening review
Next Mrs G's surgical, medical, social, and family medical history were reviewed with her as well as any preventative screenings. She stated she did commit to mammograms; most recent one last year was negative for cancer. Mrs G knew she needed a yearly diabetic eye examination but had "gotten behind" due to the pandemic and would schedule an appointment. Mrs G was up to date on her immunizations and had received both her COVID-19 vaccines.

Social review
The MC Annual Wellness Visit has a section for providers to review social factors. Mrs G had never smoked, consumed illegal drugs, or drank alcohol. She has an advanced care directive, and her son is her health care power of attorney.

Cognition assessment
An important component of the AWV requirement, a mini cognitive test is conducted. Mrs. G drew the clock without problem and remembered 2 of the 3 words given. She admitted that for the past year, she is "not remembering as well." Although her score does not warrant further dementia screening,

cognitive impairment in older adults may be due to medication side effects and depression and can be reversed or improved with treatment [5].

Depression screening

The Patient Health Questionnaire-9 depression screen was completed, as she verbalized "yes" to the second question about feeling down, depressed, or hopeless. Her screening score was 8 of 27, indicating mild depression. The NP discussed her verbalized feelings of depression and feeling bad about herself as well as her insomnia. Her recent fall and lack of exercise during the pandemic had her weakened and feeling "blue." Mrs G also stated the COVID-19 pandemic, and the social isolation had affected her a great deal. Mrs G mentioned she did not see her friends at church, and now, she was afraid to go back to church in fear of falling. Depression in the older adult is not normal and can be treated successfully when identified and treated early [3]. Loneliness is a psychosocial issue that should be considered during the AWV because there is a link between loneliness and poor health outcomes [3].

While in the home, the NP noticed a young man was in a bedroom down the hall playing video games and talking loudly in his bedroom. When asked about him Mrs G opened up and revealed that her 15-year-old grandson lives with her since his mother died 4 years ago from an overdose and his father is incarcerated. She states that her grandson has mental health "anger issues." She also told me that she is afraid to correct or discipline him in any way because he becomes irate, and she is afraid of him. Mrs G stated that her grandson sees a therapist for his mental health issues. This situation prompted a telephone call to her PCP to make him aware. She was informed that the situation along with her feelings of isolation would trigger a social work referral and she would be contacted within 24 hours by a social worker to discuss her concerns and provide resources. Ms G agreed to the referral.

Social determinants of health assessment

Underserved older adults often face disparities in healthy aging. Such disparities are likely due to individual, social, and behavioral determinants of health such as low income, limited education, social isolation, food insecurity, poor housing quality, and difficulty affording medications. These areas of concern are addressed in a Social Determinants of Health (SDOH) risk tool. New AWV models should address important root causes of poor health, such as individual, behavioral, and SDOH. Assessment of these areas has the potential to promote healthy aging among underserved seniors [6]. Mrs G verbalized no financial difficulties and has no problems paying for food, essentials, utilities, or transportation for herself or her grandson. She states she had no fear of losing her housing and no need for personal assistance.

Social isolation risk

Mrs G states she did not talk or see anyone except her grandson sometimes for days at a time. This, in combination with problems communicating with her grandson, indicated some social isolation. She said her neighbors are nice, but she does not always talk to them. Mrs G said that her son and daughter-in-law lived an hour away but did not visit because of past altercations with her grandson.

Elder mistreatment risk

Mrs G stated she felt safe at home but only because she will not say or do anything to anger her grandson. When asked about the grandson's behavior, she stated that he "yells" and "curses" at her but has never pushed or been violent toward her. Mrs G stated that if he ever did, she would call 911 for his removal from the home. The NP encouraged her to talk to the grandson's counselor who sees him for his anger issues. Before the Covid-19 pandemic, research indicated 1 in 10 older adults experienced abuse or neglect by a caregiver with only a fraction of the cases reported. An on-line US study conducted during the stay-at-home orders indicated 1 in 5 older adults reported abuse, suggesting that rate of elder abuse in the community had increased by 84% since the beginning of the pandemic. It has been noted that only a fraction of elder abuse cases are reported. Thus, providers should assess/observe for signs/symptoms that suggest the possibility of elder abuse [7]. These signs/symptoms include signs of bruising greater than 5 cm on unusual areas of the body and not over bony prominences, that is, arms, face, and back; burns inconsistent with injuries; missing medications; dehydration; malnutrition; decubitus; intraoral soft tissue injuries; patterned injuries, that is, slap or bite marks, scars, or bruises on wrists and/or ankles; and unexplained fractures [8,9].

Physical assessment

Vital signs revealed a blood pressure 140/80 and heart rate of 64. Lungs were clear. Minimal lower extremity edema was noted, and Mrs G states her feet swell toward the end of the day. She was encouraged to elevate her legs for 30 minutes at least twice daily in her recliner. The NP provided scales for her to weigh and measured her height. Mrs G's BMI was 47.8, stating it was difficult for her to lose weight because she could not walk like she did before her injury. Range of motion to her left knee was decreased but range of motion to right knee was within normal limits. No crepitus was appreciated. She did have her knee brace on and states she wears it "most of the day" but takes it off at bedtime. Dorsalis pedis pulses were palpable at +2.

At the end of the visit, the NP reviewed recommendations. Mrs G agreed for the NP to call her PCP to recommend weaning of alprazolam and starting trazadone or another antidepressant that would help lift mood and enhance sleep. It was recommended Mrs G consider taking melatonin, 5 to 10 mg, along with acetaminophen, 650 mg, at bedtime to help with sleep during this transition. It was discussed with her to reduce carbohydrates and increase vegetable intake as well as consider small servings to reduce calorie intake. She agreed to walk with a cane down the hall and back at least 5 times in a row and work to repeat the walk 3 times a day. Lastly, the NP reminded her to talk to her grandson's therapist about her fears of his aggression. She agreed to leave home and call 911 if she ever felt in danger.

Recommendations for ensuring a time-efficient Annual Wellness Visit
The 60-minute visit provides the time for a comprehensive history taking, multiple risk assessments, medication reconciliation, health screenings, and personalized planning for the prevention needed for better health and well-being. In order to keep the visit within the allotted time limit, the provider should keep on task and redirect the individual as needed in conversation. Flowing from one assessment piece to another in conversation/interview style allows the most information to be collected during the shortest amount of time. Review of prior years' AWV notes, medical history, and having supplies at hand ensure that the visit is completed in the most efficient manner.

COMPARISON OF HOME AND CLINIC SETTINGS FOR THE ANNUAL WELLNESS VISIT

The MC AWV is completed in the home by a health care provider hired by the MC complete insurance company or in the clinic by the PCP. The provider conducting the home MC AWV has the unique opportunity to personally encounter the individual and his/her home environment, enabling a closer look into needs that may not be verbalized.

Social conversation has been noted to build better relationships that enhance communication between provider and patient [8]. Sitting with the patient in his/her home provides a relaxed environment for open and honest communication. Although a home visit certainly has many benefits for both the practitioner and the patient, a clinic visit may, at times, be more appropriate or comfortable for the patient. The provider conducting the AWV in the clinic setting does have the ability to perform many of the recommended tests at the AWV time, and referred tests can be scheduled during the visit. In addition, if the patient is having an acute problem, this can be addressed and billed for with the use of modifiers, briefly discussed later. The home and clinic settings are both appropriate settings for the AWV. MC recipients may have an AWV from both PCP and by a representative of their insurance company. Choice and preference of the MC recipient is the guide for what setting is used for the AWV. In either case, the AWV is a valuable tool in attaining optimal health.

A PROACTIVE APPROACH TO ASSESSING MENTAL HEALTH AND WELL-BEING IN THE PRIMARY CARE CLINIC

Performance of the AWV is becoming more common in the primary care setting, as patients are more acclimated to the purpose of the visit. One challenge remains, that of performing a successful and complete AWV in a 1-hour time slot. A team approach with the clinic staff can help to create an efficient flow to meet the time challenges as well as the multiple tasks involved in the AWV. Reallocation of nursing resources to assist with particular areas of the AWV can free up some of the health care professional's (HCP's) time [10]. The registered nurse/licensed vocational nurse can make a previsit call to do the following:

- Update past medical/surgical/social/family/dietary histories;
- Reconcile medication lists;
- Perform falls risk;
- Complete functional ability assessment;
- Perform visual and hearing acuities;
- Conduct brief depression and cognitive impairment assessment to see if further screening is indicated;
- Provide Advance Directive/Physician Orders for Life-Sustaining Treatment (POLST) forms if indicated.

This can then be ready for the HCP to review and focus on areas of concern, as well as completing the AWV. In addition, some clinics have electronic medical eecord systems set up to allow the patient to self-complete certain aspects of the AWV.

Following is a sample case study of a patient who came to clinic for his AWV.

Mr K is a 72-year-old man, a patient at the Geriatric Primary Care Clinic. He is being managed for hypertension (controlled with losartan, 50 mg) and hyperlipidemia (controlled with use of over-the-counter Omega 3 oil supplements). He had been a caregiver for more than 2 years for his wife of 45 years, who had a diagnosis of end-stage heart failure. She passed away 8 months ago due to exacerbation of her heart condition and COVID-19 complications. She died in the hospital; her husband was not allowed to be with her during this time due to COVID-19 precautions. They have no children, but he has several supportive friends with whom he is in daily contact. Mr K presents at the clinic for a scheduled AWV; his last AWV was 1 year ago (Box 2).

Box 2: Mr K's Annual Wellness Visit 1 year ago

Physical Assessment:

- BMI: stable at 26
- Colorectal screening, prostate screening, electrocardiogram all within functional limits
- Continent of urine, without nocturia
- No falls or fear of falling
- ADL/IADL screenings indicated he physically and functionally does not require assistance with any household/personal care tasks and therefore independent

Psychosocial Screening

- PHQ-2 score was 0/2; Geriatric Depression Scale (GDS) and anxiety scales were both negative
- Saint Louis University Mental Status (SLUMS) cognitive screening score was 29/30
- Denied use of tobacco, alcohol, or recreational substance use or abuse
- Suicide screening was negative; domestic abuse screening negative
- Safety screening: owns handguns, which are stored under lock and key; no fear of his safety in his home environment

Depression screening is key in Mr K's AWV this year, due to the loss of his spouse. Although the screening is an essential task during an initial AWV [3], subsequent screenings would be beneficial to older adults who will often experience sudden and significant changes in their lives. Older adults often present with other than the usual symptoms of depression, such as change in cognitive function, loss of interest or pleasure in life, and increasing isolation and loneliness [2]. These changes may then lead to sleep disorders, decreased appetite, weight loss, and possible frailty syndrome. In this situation, the NP is anticipating a decline in some, if not all of the screenings, compared with Mr K's previous AWV's results (Box 3).

Mr K has had a significant change in several areas of his psychosocial screenings that indicate a high probability of depression, likely precipitated by the loss of his wife. Results of the adverse findings of the screenings were communicated to the patient so that he could understand the provider's concerns because of the physical and psychosocial changes the patient has had since the death of his wife. In further discussion with the patient, he related he was not able to attend to her at the time of her death in the hospital and was isolated from family and friends due to COVID-19 restrictions. Further complicating the situation, he was unable to have a memorial service/funeral due to COVID-19 restrictions. Before her death, he was happy to cook and prepare meals for them both. He relates there is no use cooking "just for

---

Box 3: Mr K's current Annual Wellness Visit

Physical Assessments:

- BMI dropped to 22
- Colorectal screening not due for 3 years
- Evaluation of ADL/IADL indicates he is physically and functionally able to care for himself independently.
- No falls in 12 months; does not fear falling

Psychosocial Screening:

- SLUMS score 26/30, with decrease in areas of recent memory, concentration (indicates mild cognitive disorder)
- PHQ-9 score of 5/9 (indicates depression)
- General Anxiety Disorder-7 score of 9 (indicates mild anxiety)
- GDS scale 7/15 (indicates depression)
- Use of tobacco, alcohol, and recreation drugs: negative
- Ages & Stages Questionnaires suicide screening tool negative for feelings of suicide
- Mini Nutritional Assessment-Short Form (MNA-SF) is performed due to significant decrease in BMI over the past year, showing the patient is at risk for malnutrition

one person," and he really does not have an appetite. He has had his COVID-19 vaccinations and can attend activities with friends, but has declined to do so, related to poor motivation to get out of his home. All indicators point to the potential for development of prolonged grief with adjustment disorder, which could then lead to development of significant health and mental wellness issues.

PLANNING FOR CARE TO ENHANCE WELL-BEING BASED ON THE ANNUAL WELLNESS VISIT

The question to be asked at the conclusion of the AWV is whether the patient can be followed-up later to treat his depression or if the depression should be treated before he leaves the clinic. Although AMV focuses on the preventive problems, Mr K has shown evidence of a current problem that he is experiencing and should be treated accordingly as an acute situation. If an acute problem arises that needs to be addressed during the AWV, then a modifier to the billing (such as modifier-25) would be allowed, and the additional evaluation/management of the condition would be billed according to the codes assigned for these types of visits [1]. For further clarification, correspondence with the clinic's billing manager may be of great benefit for this situation.

Recommendations for Mr K would include laboratory work to determine if any pathologic problem is causing his depression and decreased cognition. A nutritionist consult would also be recommended for him, to assist in making healthy choices and for healthy cooking for one. Social work evaluation to assist in social determinations and barriers to care for his mental health issues is essential to getting Mr K back to a more optimal state of health. Recommendations for grief support groups in the community may also be of particular benefit.

Discussion with Mr K as to whether to start antidepressant medications should also happen at this time. Expectations of the medications, adverse and desired effects, and potential benefit versus risks should be well delineated at this time. It may be that Mr K wants to wait and see if nonpharmacological interventions may be of benefit. These interventions may include the following:

- Cognitive behavioral therapy
- Mindfulness interventions
- Music therapy
- Yoga/Tai Chi
- Connection with a grief support group or hospice for after-care

The desires of the patient are imperative as to the success of the treatment. Follow-up in 2 to 4 weeks from this visit would be most desirable to evaluate treatment modalities.

Subtle changes in the screenings that occurred during the AWV led to the diagnosis of depression. It is important to note he had not been in the clinic since the death of his wife, although he was having weight loss, sleep problems, and some mild cognitive impairment. These issues did not indicate a problem necessarily to him but because of the benefit of the AWV, he was evaluated and treated expeditiously before more problems could occur. When changes do not readily occur, or are only slight in severity, the patient may not see the changes as a problem, as in this case. The benefits of the AWV are substantiated by this example. NP, as advocates and educators for improved outcomes in preventative care, are uniquely able to assist patients such as Mr K in developing proactive wellness prevention before health damage worsens or becomes irreversible.

Although overall participation in AWV rates have not been as great as hoped, providers recognize these visits are valuable in providing important preventative services and closing quality measure gaps. MC complete insurance programs offer recipients incentives to complete the AWV to improve disease prevention and close gaps in care. Within the primary care clinic setting, the challenge remaining is in increasing the number of participations in AWV without overburdening the provider, practice, and electronic health record capabilities and related costs [1]. NPs are well positioned to incorporate the goals of the AWV for their older patients into their practice. By developing and/or updating a personalized prevention plan, striving toward preventing disease and disability based on current health and risk factors of each patient, and then educating the patient on health, advance directives, and prevention of disease, mutual goals can be set to promote the older adult's mental health and well-being [11]. Nurse practitioners are challenged to incorporate the data collected during the AWV throughout the year, working collaboratively with their patients to ensure that goals toward optimal mental health are attained [12].

CLINICS CARE POINTS

- During the annual Medicare Wellness Exam, the nurse practitioner should first review the prior history, approach the patient with no bias and formulate a mutual plan with the patient.

References
[1] Cuenca AE, Kapsner S. Medicare wellness visits: reassessing their value to your patients and your practice. Fam Pract Manag 2019;26(2):25–30.
[2] Hain DJ. The CMS Annual Wellness Visit: bridging the gap. Nurse Pract 2014;39(7):18–27.
[3] Pfoh E, Mojtabai R, Bailey J, et al. Impact of medicare annual wellness visits on uptake of depression screening. Psychiatr Serv 2015;66(11):1207–12.
[4] Medicare Wellness Visits. Available at: https://www.cms.gov/Outreach-and-(wellness-visits.html November 23, 2021.
[5] Assessing Cognitive Impairment in Older Adults. Available at: https://www.nia.nih.gov/health/assessing-cognitive-impairment-older-patients November 23, 2021.
[6] Tipirneni R, Ganguli I, Ayanian JZ, et al. Reducing disparities in healthy aging through an enhanced medicare annual wellness visit. Public Policy Aging Rep 2019;29(1):26–32.
[7] Chang E-S, Levy BR. High Prevalence of Elder Abuse During the COVID-19 pandemic: risk and resilience factors. Am J Geriatr Psychiatry 2021;66(11):1152–9.
[8] Elder Abuse. Available at: https://www.who.int/news-room/fact-sheets/detail/elder-abuse November 28, 2021.

[9] Parish AL. Opportunities for the advanced practice nurse in improving the wellbeing of older adults during the COVID-19 pandemic. Geriatr Nurs 2021;42(2):605–7.

[10] Cuenca AE. Making medicare wellness visits work in practice. Fam Pract Manag 2012;19(5):11–6.

[11] Camacho F, Yao NA, Anderson R. The effectiveness of medicare wellness visits in accessing preventive screening. J Prim Care Community Health 2017;8(4):247–55.

[12] Simpson V, Edwards N, Kovich M. Conversations about wellness: A qualitative analysis of patient narratives post annual wellness visit. Geriatr Nurs 2021;42(3):681–6.

Basic Considerations for Understanding and Treating Delirium Psychosis in Older Adults

Cecilia A. Nwogu, DNP, GNP-BC, PMHNP[a],*,
Linda J. Keilman, DNP, GNP-BC, FAANP[b],
George Byron Peraza-Smith, DNP, APRN-C, GNP-BC, GS-C, FAANP[c],
Pamela Z. Cacchione, PhD, CRNP, BC, FSGA, FAAN[d],
Sharon Bronner, DNP, GNP-BC, ACHPN[e],
Karen Devereaux Melillo, PhD, A-GNP-C, FAANP, FGSA[f],
Amy M. Lewitz, MS, APRN, PMHCNS[g],
Tamatha Arms, PhD, DNP, PMHNP-BC, NP-C[h],
Melodee Harris, PhD, RN, FAAN[i]

[a]CobbWest Internal Medicine Associates, 848 Hiram Acworth Hwy, Bldg 200, Ste A, Hiram GA, 30141; [b]Michigan State University, College of Nursing, 1355 Bogue Street, A126 Life Science Building, East Lansing, MI 48824-1317, USA; [c]South University, 709 Mall Boulevard, Savannah, GA 31406, USA; [d]University of Pennsylvania, School of Nursing, 418 Curie Boulevard, Philadelphia, PA 19104-4217, USA; [e]Centers Health Care, 1540 Tomlinson Avenue, Bronx, NY 10461, USA; [f]Solomont School of Nursing, Zuckerberg College of Health Sciences University of Massachusetts Lowell, Health and Social Sciences Building, Suite 200, 113 Wilder Street, Lowell, MA, USA; [g]6942 North Kilpatrick, Lincolnwood, IL 60712, USA; [h]UNCW CHHS School of Nursing, Wilmington, NC, USA; [i]University of Arkansas for Medical Sciences, College of Nursing, 4301 West Markham Street, Slot #529, Little Rock, AR 72205, USA

Keywords
• Delirium • Psychosis • Delirium superimposed on dementia

Key points
• Delirium is characterized as an acute confusional state resulting from comprehensive impairment in cognitive function. Older age is a risk factor for delirium.

Continued

Corresponding author. E-mail address: adhc.inc@gmail.com

https://doi.org/10.1016/j.yfpn.2021.12.003
2589-420X/22/

Continued

- Delirium can present as hypoactive or hyperactive states and may fluctuate between the two.
- Dementia and delirium are often co-occurring conditions. Dementia is a risk factor for delirium. Delirium superimposed on dementia is not due to a single factor.
- Charles Bonnet syndrome is an atypical cause of visual hallucinations owing to poor visual acuity often worse than 20/60.
- Terminal delirium occurs at the end-of-life. Death bed visions are typically not fearful to the older adult but are a concern for family.

OVERVIEW

Delirium is characterized as an acute confusional state resulting from comprehensive impairment in cognitive function [1,2]. Older age is a risk factor for delirium and is especially common after surgeries [2,3]. Delirium is a complex syndrome that should be treated as a medical emergency [4,5,6]. Delayed or untreated delirium may result in permanent brain damage [3,7]. Prevention of delirium is always the best course of action [4,6,8]. Despite best efforts, delirium can still occur. Early diagnosis and treatment are paramount [6]. The following case studies provide brief, real-life scenarios that focus on atypical late-life psychosis associated with delirium that may be encountered in the primary care setting. The pathophysiology, assessment, diagnosis, treatment, and preventive measures related to these presentations are also explored. The 3 specific atypical presentations are (1) delirium superimposed on dementia, (2) Charles Bonnet syndrome (CBS), and (3) end-of-life (EOL) psychosis.

DEFINITION

The American Psychiatric Association's fifth edition of the *Diagnostic and Statistical Manual of Mental Disorders (DSM-5)* [1] revised the diagnostic criteria for delirium (Box 1). Delirium can present as hypoactive or hyperactive states and may fluctuate between the two [1].

PATHOPHYSIOLOGY

The pathogenesis of delirium is not well understood [4,9], especially with the coexistence of psychosis [2,3]. Delirium is described by widespread dysfunction, inflammation, and structural abnormalities within the blood-brain barrier. It is thought that neurotransmitters may play an important role in the cause of delirium [9,10]. The key to determining the pathogenesis of delirium is to differentiate the signs and symptoms from psychosis and delirium and identify the underlying potential causes [2,3,6].

ASSESSMENT FINDINGS

High rates of unrecognized delirium by providers and nurses [6] emphasize the importance of screening for delirium. The Confusion Assessment Method

> **Box 1: *Diagnostic Criteria***
>
> A. A disturbance in attention (i.e., reduced ability to direct, focus, sustain, and shift attention) and awareness (reduced orientation to the environment).
>
> B. The disturbance develops over a short period of time (usually hours to a few days), represents a change from baseline attention and awareness, and tends to fluctuate in severity during the course of a day.
>
> C. An additional disturbance in cognition (e.g., memory deficit, disorientation, language, visuospatial ability, or perception).
>
> D. The disturbances in Criteria A and C are not better explained by another pre-existing, established, or evolving neurocognitive disorder and do not occur in the context of a severely reduced level of arousal, such as coma.
>
> E. There is evidence from the history, physical examination, or laboratory findings that the disturbance is a direct physiological consequence of another medical condition, substance intoxication or withdrawal (i.e., due to a drug of abuse or to a medication), or exposure to a toxin, or is due to multiple etiologies.
>
> *Specify whether:*
>
> **Substance intoxication delirium**: This diagnosis should be made instead of substance intoxication when the symptoms in Criteria A and C predominate in the clinical picture and when they are sufficiently severe to warrant clinical attention.
>
> *Reprinted with permission from* the Diagnostic and Statistical Manual of Mental Disorders, Fifth Edition, (Copyright © 2013). American Psychiatric Association. All Rights Reserved.

(CAM) is a common assessment tool. The CAM is based on the *DSM-IV* criteria for delirium. The CAM is a useful tool for screening and assessing for delirium [11]. The CAM identifies the following 4 distinguishing features from dementia or other cognitive impairments:

1. Acute onset or fluctuating course
2. Inattention
3. Disorganized thinking
4. Altered levels of consciousness

TREATMENT

The Yale Delirium Prevention Trial showed a decrease of delirium from 15% to 9% by targeting the following 6 factors [12]:

1. Orientation
2. Early mobilization
3. Medication reconciliation
4. Sleep-wake cycle preservation
5. Sensory impairment
6. Dehydration

Once delirium is diagnosed, treatment needs to begin right away. Treatment should be aimed at the underlying cause of the delirium and may be multifactorial. Medications used to treat delirium are used off-label. The lowest dose of medications that is absolutely needed should be used, and medications should be weaned as soon as appropriate to do so.

NONPHARMACOLOGIC TREATMENT

Nurses have more control over the patient environment than medications. A calm, relaxing environment is important for delirium prevention [3]. The environment should be well-lit during the day and lighting should be reduced at night to aid in a proper sleep/wake cycle [13]. Orientation to time and place, cognitive stimulation, hydration, and early mobilization are effective strategies for delirium prevention [3,6]. Eliminating urinary catheters and intravenous lines is an important intervention to control delirium [4]. Physical restraints should be avoided [4].

CASE STUDIES

All delirium is not the same. The characteristics and treatment of delirium must be individualized. The following case studies explain atypical presentations of delirium in older adults and provide guidance for assessment, diagnosing, and treatment options. The 3 case studies are examples of older adults with delirium superimposed on dementia, CBS, and terminal delirium.

Delirium superimposed on dementia case study: Mr James is a 79-year-old man residing in a memory care unit since it opened 7 years ago, longer than most of the other residents. He is prescribed an acetylcholinesterase inhibitor. Mr James has multiple comorbid conditions and medication treatments for diabetes, dyslipidemia, coronary artery disease, stage 3 chronic kidney failure, and pulmonary hypertension (HTN).

Mr James has a unique sense of humor and typically a gentle, calm nature. He owned a small café that was open for breakfast for more than 45 years before he retired. He loves to eat! The staff typically bring extra treats that they know Mr James likes. Mr James enjoys the attention and is cooperative with care. Compared with the other residents, Mr James is physically strong and can manage activities of daily living with assistance.

Over the past 2 weeks, the nursing assistants report that something is not right. During evening meals, Mr James was increasingly angry, hypervigilant with difficulty focusing attention, and was easily distracted. He refused to eat and alleged the staff poisoned his food. He is more incontinent and cannot wear shoes due to pedal edema. Mr James started to experience new onset nighttime restlessness, daytime napping, and wandering in and out of rooms looking for potato chips.

Over the next few days, the frequency of argumentative confrontations and raising his fist to other residents continued to escalate. While wandering aimlessly around the unit, he had a resident-to-resident physical encounter. The altercation with another resident in the dining room was over snacks that Mr James thought belonged to him. The nursing staff is concerned that Mr James will be discharged from the unit to keep other residents safe.

The advanced practice registered nurse (APRN) who assessed Mr James recognized sudden changes from being calm and easily redirected that progressed to anger and frustration. Using the CAM screening tool, the APRN noted Mr James scored positive in all 4 features for delirium:

- *Feature 1: Acute onset.* Mr James' behavior had changed quickly; he became quick to anger and was suspicious of staff and residents.
- *Feature 2: Inattention.* Mr James' speech became tangential; he struggled to stay on topic.
- *Feature 3: Disorganized thinking.* Mr James would mumble to himself with illogical and disorganized thoughts.
- *Feature 4: Altered level of consciousness.* Mr James was hypervigilant and wandered aimlessly around the unit and wandered into other residents' rooms.

In this case study, the diagnosis is delirium superimposed on dementia. Dementia and delirium are often comorbid conditions [6]. Dementia is a risk factor for delirium [3]. The cause of delirium superimposed on dementia in this scenario is not due to a single factor. The differential diagnoses include hyperglycemia, heart failure, or urinary tract infection (UTI). The rounding APRN found that Mr James' blood glucose levels were elevated. Metformin had been discontinued several weeks previously related to low creatinine clearance. The evening nurse used the sliding scale and communicated with the on-call provider for elevated glucose higher than 400; unfortunately, the APRN most knowledgeable about Mr James was on vacation, and the report was missed on the daytime shift.

The APRN ordered a comprehensive metabolic panel to determine electrolyte imbalance, hemoglobin A_{1c}, brain-type natriuretic peptide, complete blood count, and urinalysis with culture and sensitivity. Based on the blood work, Mr James' Levemir, a long-acting insulin, was adjusted to manage nighttime blood sugar fluctuations to avoid use of short-acting sliding scale insulin. He had a UTI and was prescribed an antibiotic. Within 5 days, Mr James' blood sugars were under control. His furosemide was increased for 3 days, and sodium intake was monitored closely. He was prescribed melatonin 3 mg at bedtime and began to sleep better after 7 days. Mr James' amiable baseline personality returned.

Family continued to bring snacks, but limited candy bars and cookies. The evening, nighttime, and weekend staff were educated to anticipate Mr James' needs. The daytime staff were educated to help decrease daytime napping and increase engaging Mr James in outside activities and games on the memory unit.

CBS case study: Mr Jones is a 78-year-old African American man who is a member of a Program of All-Inclusive Care for the Elderly (PACE). He has a history of HTN, type 2 diabetes, osteoarthritis, and diabetic retinopathy in both eyes. He scores 26/30 on the Mini Mental Status Examination [14] and 4/28 on his Patient Health Questionnaire-9 [15]. He reports to his primary care Nurse Practitioner (NP) that over the last several weeks he has been experiencing "visions" of Italian men in suits with hats on. He reports that they smile at him but never say anything; then they disappear. He knows they are not real. They do not scare him. He just wants to make sure he is not going "crazy!" The NP starts a delirium workup because the hallucinations are new. The delirium workup was negative. She referred Mr Jones to ophthalmology and the mental health team at the PACE Center. The mental health team was aware of CBS, and this disorder was later confirmed by the ophthalmologist. The mental health APRN started cognitive behavioral therapy (CBT) with Mr Jones. He completed 6 weeks of weekly CBT with good results. The hallucinations did not resolve, but

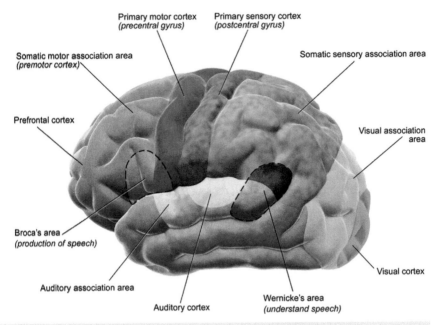

Fig. 1. Visual association and visual cortex diagram. (*Adapted from* Blausen.com staff (2014). "Medical gallery of Blausen Medical 2014". WikiJournal of Medicine 1 (2). https://doi.org/10.15347/wjm/2014.010. ISSN 2002-4436; CC BY 3.0)

Mr Jones was not disturbed by them and used the techniques he learned in CBT to address his daily hallucinations.

An atypical cause of visual hallucinations includes CBS. Persons with bilateral visual impairment may present with visual hallucinations that are either persistent or recurrent during a clear state of consciousness [16]. This is due to spontaneous activity in the extrastriate visual cortex [17] in areas of the brain responsible for processing features of some visual information (Fig. 1).

The most common age range for the development of CBS is between ages 70 and 85 years [18]. Ten percent to 13% of individuals with bilateral visual acuity worse than 20/60 are reported to have such visual hallucinations [19].

CBS was first identified in the 1760s by Charles Bonnet [20], and the most used diagnostic criteria were described by Gold and Rabins [16]. These criteria include the following:

- Persons with CBS report seeing repeating patterns of lines or other geometric shapes
- Mountains or waterfalls
- People, animals, or insects
- People dressed in costume from an earlier time

- Imaginary creatures

The hallucinations may be stationary or mobile. The hallucinations are often vivid in color but may also appear in black and white, lasting seconds to hours [21].

The person's insight is fully or partially intact. The person is without primary or secondary delusions, or hallucinations in other modalities [16,22]. The differential for CBS includes the following:

- Schizophrenia
- Bipolar disorder
- Lewy body dementia
- Parkinson disease
- Substance misuse versus medication causes [22]

Treatment for CBS includes patient and family education that these visual hallucinations are not a sign of mental illness or dementia [20]. This reassurance is often all patients and families need to address and treat these nonthreatening visual hallucinations. CBT can be used to address the distress that can be experienced from the visual hallucinations. If reassurance is not sufficient, medication may decrease the frequency of the visual hallucinations. However, the risk and benefits of medication therapy should be weighed carefully. If the trial of medications is not helpful, they should be discontinued. Medication management for hallucinations that are distressing include antipsychotics, anticonvulsants, and selective serotonin reuptake inhibitors [18].

Terminal psychosis (delirium) at the EOL case study: A.R. is an 81-year-old man who was living in a skilled nursing facility (SNF) for 9 years. His wife lives out in the community with her daughter's family (this is his second marriage). A.R. has one son and one daughter. In the last 6 months, the patient had frequent falls due to forgetting he could not walk any longer and increased confusion after 1500 hours (3:00 PM). He has diagnoses of dementia, HTN, and diastolic heart failure and is on palliative care. His medications include the following: lisinopril 5 mg by mouth daily, vitamin D 1000 IU by mouth daily, calcium 500 mg by mouth twice a day with meals, and ferrous sulfate 325 mg by mouth daily. He suddenly developed coughing without mucus production and a decreased appetite. A chest radiograph revealed bilateral infiltrates in the bilateral lower lobes. A.R. was prescribed Rocephin 1 g via an intravenous route, Proventil every 6 hours, cough medicine, and increased oral fluids.

After 3 days, the certified nursing assistant (CNA) reported to the APRN that the patient was talking in Spanish about him seeing his mother soon and that he misses her so much. The CNA was very concerned and started to be tearful. Support was given to the nursing staff and CNA; education was provided on EOL psychosis or terminal psychosis. Three days later, A.R. died of pneumonia. A nebulizer was not used in the SNF because of the presence of the COVID-19 pandemic and the potential to spread the virus via aerosol from nebulization.

Delirium is a serious cognitive disorder that is often missed at the EOL. *Terminal delirium* (psychosis) is not a distinct diagnosis, although it is a commonly used phrase. It implies delirium in a patient in the final days or weeks of life, where treatment of the underlying cause is impossible to reverse.

Terminal agitation or restlessness can be defined as agitated delirium with cognitive impairment. The main symptoms are agitation, myoclonic jerks or twitching, irritability, and impaired consciousness [23–25]. Other symptoms include hallucinations, paranoia, confusion, and disorientation. Terminal delirium symptoms, such as agitation and restlessness, have been reported to be the most difficult EOL symptoms to manage.

CAUSES OF TERMINAL PSYCHOSIS

Terminal psychosis or terminal delirium occurs at the EOL and can be a burden to families and caregivers. The last 3 to 7 days of life can be a challenge for family harmony. Common symptoms may include, but are not limited to, difficulty communicating, memory disorganization, and disorientation. Identification of behavioral symptoms and terminal psychosis is essential to help maintain older adults' comfort and promote quality of life (QOL).

SUBTYPES OF DELIRIUM

Visions are sometimes associated with delirium at the EOL. As the older adult approaches death, visions of people who have died in the past, known as deathbed visions, may occur. The older adult sees these individuals or family members as *guides* assisting in the transition from life to death [23]. Deathbed visions have been defined as an unexplained experience or experiences or coincidental occurrence or occurrences that take place when approaching death [26]. The experiential phenomena are not fearful. The older adult is usually calm, can focus attention to the vision [23], and generally enjoys these experiences.

Another delirium subtype associated with the EOL is nearing death awareness (NDA). NDA is a term used to describe a dying person's experiences of the process and broadly refers to a variety of experiences such as EOL dreams or visions. The recognition of NDA requires attentive listening. The content of NDA often will vary based on cultural background.

ASSESSMENT

A comprehensive assessment, including physical, psychosocial, and spiritual assessment, is needed. A standard workup can help to rule out nonpsychiatric causes of psychosis, as well as some additional tests if clinically necessary. These may include the following:

- Complete blood count
- Metabolic panel
- Urinalysis
- Urine cultures

- Thyroid-stimulating hormone, T3, T3
- Liver function
- Vitamin B12
- HIV
- Computed tomography scan or MRI [4]

PREVENTION AND INTERVENTION IN TERMINAL PSYCHOSIS

Tertiary prevention for terminal psychosis focuses on the limitation of disability and suffering by addressing the findings of a root cause. Anticipation of a patient's decline can lead the clinician to consult with palliative/hospice care services. Referral for psychotherapy to focus on coping and defense mechanisms can help reduce the risk for decompensation and psychosis. For older adults who have not responded to psychosocial interventions, low-dose antipsychotics and/or anxiolytics are indicated for relief of severe emotional distress and/or concurrent agitation. Haloperidol should be reserved for emergency use during an acute bout of psychosis. The guiding dosing principle is to start low and go slow. Intervention is aimed at maintaining comfort while assuring safety for the patient with terminal psychosis.

INTERVENTION

The application of evidence-based practice guidelines by an interdisciplinary team is essential for optimal care of older adults with terminal delirium. The management of delirium in the final hours and days of life should make every effort to address the safety and presenting symptoms [23]. Nonpharmacologic approaches may be beneficial to address the deathbed phenomena experiences. The APRN should reframe the experiences and acknowledge the importance of guiding loved ones to say good-bye.

SUMMARY

Older adults are thriving and optimally aging with mental and chronic illnesses. Some older adults adapt to psychosis that accompanies serious and persistent mental illness with an increase in psychosocial interactions and improved self-reported well-being [27]. Nurses are most likely to encounter older adults with these atypical presentations of delirium psychosis across all care settings. Despite the biomarkers associated with accelerated biological aging and increasing vulnerability to delirium psychosis associated with chronic illnesses and premature mortality rates [28], a good number of older adults are surviving with mental conditions and aging optimally.

What is aging optimally? Optimal aging is an optimistic, positive paradigm that may foster positive perceptions of aging among students when compared with a decay and decline paradigm. Optimal aging focuses on the development of meaningful interventions that improve QOL [29]. Negative attitudes toward older adults (often referred to as ageism) can lead to a decrease in the quality of care.

Ageism can promote misdiagnosis, inappropriate care for and treatment of specific conditions, polypharmacy, and less aggressive or mutual goal setting [30,31].

Changing attitudes, implementing a positive approach to older adults, and recognition of delirium psychosis contribute to optimal aging. Gerontological nurses need the expertise to care for older adults with psychosis and reach beyond the illness to decrease stigma. The mere fact that many marginalized older adults with psychosis are beginning to decrease the odds for increased mortality and mental health disparities is phenomenal. Gerontological nurses must recognize the delirium psychosis, but it is the person inside the older adults who inspires resiliency.

Disclosure
The authors have no disclosures.

References

[1] American Psychiatric Association. Diagnostic and statistical manual of mental disorders. 5th edition. American Psychiatric Publishing; 2013 DSM-V, doi-org.db29.linccweb.org/10.1176/.

[2] Wilson JE, Mart MF, Cunningham C, et al. Delirium. Nat Rev Dis Primers 2020;6:90; https://doi.org/10.1038/s41572-020-00223-4.

[3] Inouye SK, Westendorp RG, Saczynski JS. Delirium in elderly people. Lancet (London, England) 2014;383(9920):911–22.

[4] Wan M, Chase JM. Delirium in older adults: diagnosis, prevention, and treatment. BCMJ 2017;59(3):156–70.

[5] Oh ES, Fong TG, Hshieh TT, et al. Delirium in older persons: advances in diagnosis and treatment. JAMA 2017;318(12):1161–74.

[6] Ospina JP, King F, Madva E, et al. Epidemiology, Mechanisms, Diagnosis and Treatment of Delirium: A Narrative Review. Clin Med Ther 2020;1:1; https://doi.org/10.24983/scitemed.cmt.2018.00085.

[7] Fong TG, Davis D, Growdon ME, et al. The interface between delirium and dementia in elderly adults. Lancet Neurol 2015;14(8):823–32.

[8] Bellelli G, Brathwaite JS, Mazzola P. Delirium: a marker of vulnerability in older people. Front Aging Neurosci 2021;13:626127; https://doi.org/10.3389/fnagi.2021.626127.

[9] Hshieh TT, Inouye SK, Oh ES. Delirium in the elderly. Psychiatr Clin N Am 2018;41:1–17.

[10] Mulkey MA, Hardin SR, Olson DM, et al. Pathophysiology review: seven neurotransmitters associated with delirium. Clin Nurse specialist CNS 2018;32(4):195–211.

[11] Wei LA, Fearing MA, Sternberg EJ, et al. The confusion assessment method: a systematic review of current usage. J Am Geriatr Soc 2008;56:823–30.

[12] Inouye SK, Bogardus ST Jr, Charpentier PA, Leo-Summers L, Acampora D, Holford TR, Cooney LM Jr, et al. A multicomponent intervention to prevent delirium in hospitalized older patients. N Engl J Med 1999 Mar 4;340(9):669–76; https://doi.org/10.1056/NELM199903043400901, PMID:10053175.

[13] Stahl SM, Morrisette DA. Stahl's illustrated sleep and wake disorders. Cambridge University Press; 2016.

[14] Folstein MF, Folstein SE, McHugh PR. Mini-mental state": a practical method for grading the cognitive state of patients for the clinician. J Psychiatr Res 1975;12:189–98.

[15] Kroenke K, Spitzer R, Williams J. The PHQ-9 validity of a brief depression severity measure. J Gen Intern Med 2001;16:606–13.

[16] Gold K, Rabins PV. Isolated visual hallucinations and the Charles Bonnet syndrome: a review of the literature and presentation of six cases. Comp Psychiatry 1989;30(1):90–8.

[17] Minakaran N, Soorma T, Beronstein AM, et al. Charles Bonnet syndrome and periodic alternating nystagmus. Neurology 2019;92:e1072–5.

[18] Pelak, VS. Visual release hallucinations (Charles Bonnet syndrome.) UpToDate Available at: www.uptodate.com. Accessed June 23, 2021.

[19] Mentes JC, Bail JK. Psychosis in older adults. In: Melillo KD, Houde SC, editors. Geropsychiatric and mental health nursing. 2nd edition. JB Learning; 2011. p. 203–25.

[20] Pang L. Hallucinations experienced by visually impaired: Charles Bonnet syndrome. Optom Vis Sci 2016;93(12):1466–78.

[21] Porter D. What is Charles Bonnet syndrome? Eye health A-Z for public & patients. American Academy of Ophthalmology. Available at: https://www.aao.org/eye-health/diseases/what-is-charles-bonnet-syndrome.

[22] Russel g, Harper R, Allen H, et al. Cognitive impairment and Charles Bonnet syndrome prospective study. Int. J Geriatr Psychiatry 2018;33:39–46.

[23] Curtis L. Deathbed visions: social workers' experiences, perspectives, therapeutic responses, and direction for practice. Master of Social Work Clinical Research Papers 2012 17. Available at: https://sophia.stkate.edu/msw_papers/17.

[24] Ferrell B, Coyle N, Paice JA. Oxford textbook of palliative nursing. 4th edition 2015. p. 388–91.

[25] Mazzarino-Willett A. Deathbed phenomena: its role in peaceful death and terminal restlessness. Am J Hosp Palliat Care 2010;27(2):127–33.

[26] Chevrolet JC, Jolliet P. Clinical review: agitation and delirium in the critically ill–significance and management. Crit Care 2007;11(3):214.

[27] Jeste D, Peschin S, Buckwalter K, et al. Promoting wellness in older adults with mental illness and substance use disorders: call to action to all stakeholders. Am J Geriatr Psychiatry 2018;26(6):617–30; https://doi.org/10.1016/j.jagp.2018.03.011. Available at:.

[28] Nguyen TT, Eyler LT, Jeste DV. Systemic biomarkers of accelerated aging in schizophrenia: a critical review and future directions. Schizophrenia Bull 2018;44(2):398–408; https://doi.org/10.1093/schbul/sbx069. Available at:.

[29] Avers D. Infusing an optimal aging paradigm into an entry-level geriatrics course. Phys Ther Edu 2014;28(2):22–34.

[30] Eymard AS, Douglas DH. Ageism among health care providers and interventions to improve their attitudes toward older adults: an integrative review. J Gerontol Nurs 2012;38(5):26–35; https://doi.org/10.1016/j.jagp.2018.03.011. Available at:.

[31] Liu YE, Norman IJ, While AE. Nurses' attitudes towards older people: a systematic review. Int J Nurs Stud 2012;50:1271–82.

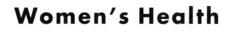

Women's Health

Integrating Behavioral Health into Primary Care for Women

Jenna Smith, LCSW, MSSW[a],
Candice Vaden, MSN, WHNP-BC, AGPCNP-BC[b],*,
Willis Smith, MSN, PMHNP-BC, LPC[c],
Christian Ketel, DNP, RN[a]

[a]Vanderbilt University School of Nursing, 2611 West End Avenue, Suite 380, Nashville, TN 37203, USA; [b]Vanderbilt Midwives Melrose, 2410 8th Avenue, South Nashville, TN 37204, USA; [c]Marin Community Clinics, 3100 Redwood Boulevard, Novato, CA 94947, USA

Keywords

- Women's health • Depression • Midwife • Integrated behavioral health
- Primary care

Key points

- Integrating behavioral health into women's health practices is beneficial to both the patients and providers based on research data
- Patients are at higher risk of mood disorder exacerbation during the perinatal time period, especially those with a previous history of a mood disorder.
- Integrating behavioral health into clinic settings provides a higher rate of success for patients with behavioral health needs than traditional care.
- Routine screening of depression and anxiety with validated tools increases provider identification of patients in need of behavioral health care.
- Easy collaboration with the behavioral health team increases provider comfort with treating mental illness.

INTRODUCTION

Mental health disorders are prevalent and rising across the United States [1]. Often these disorders are left unidentified and untreated by non–mental health care providers owing to a long-standing, systematic, and unreasonable separation of physical and mental health services in day-to-day practice [2]. The

*Corresponding author. 2410 8th Avenue South, Nashville, TN 37204, USA *E-mail address:* Candice.vaden@vumc.org

https://doi.org/10.1016/j.yfpn.2021.12.004

consequences of this systematic separation between mind and body is that it is the antithesis of person-centered, high-quality health care. Separating mental and physical health leads to a disjointed situation for both the patient and the health care system. Over the past decade, there has been a reversal in this strictly categorical way of thinking about mental health care as it relates to physical or overall health. By integrating behavioral health services back into physical health systems, health systems are achieving better overall health outcomes [3]. This article builds the case for integrating behavioral health care into women's health practices using evidence from the literature, as well as one clinical site's experience of implementing a program of integrated behavioral health into a women's health practice using the collaborative care model (CoCM). Integrating behavioral health into organizations and practices is not only possible, but a necessary part of providing truly person-centered, holistic care to those served.

PREVALENCE OF MOOD DISORDERS

According to the National Alliance on Mental Illness, during 2019, mental illness affected as many as 21% of all adults (51.5 million people) in the United States [1]. That includes 48 million adults living with anxiety disorders and 19.4 million living with some form of depressive disorder [1]. Although this situation is concerning, it is also estimated that 5% of the general adult population lives with a serious mental illness (schizophrenia, bipolar disorder, major depression, etc) [1]. By large measure, anxiety and depression disorders are the most commonly diagnosed mental health disorders in the United States. It is reported that 19.1% of the adult population in the United States experience some level of abnormal or persistent anxiety; although often co-occurring, depressive disorders are the second most prevalent mental health disorders in the United States, with 7.8% of adults experiencing at least 1 major depressive episode in their lives [1]. Additionally, post-traumatic stress disorder and obsessive–compulsive disorder are estimated to be prevalent in at least 3.6% and 1.2%, respectively, of the general adult population [1].

Overall, approximately 21% of the adult population in the United States is affected by a known diagnosis of mental illness. This has ramifications beyond both physical and mental health. According to the American Psychiatric Association, mental health disorders often lead to social and physical impairments, decreased functionality, and difficulty with employment [4]. This situation equates to a loss of working days that can reach as high as 12 billion days lost owing to mental illness every year, resulting in approximately $16 trillion lost by 2030 [5]. The disturbing reality is these data only represents those with identified mental health disorders. The true impact of mental health in the United States is likely underrepresented by these values.

SPECIFIC CONCERNS FOR WOMEN'S HEALTH AND PRIMARY CARE

It is important to note that women (particularly in the perinatal period) are twice as likely as men to be diagnosed with anxiety or depression [6]. Unique biological factors are encountered by women that may contribute to this increased prevalence. These unique factors include (but are not limited to): premenstrual syndrome, premenstrual dysphoric disorder, pregnancy, postpartum state, and perimenopause [6] (Table 1). According to one report by the Centers for Disease Control and Prevention, at least 10% of women in the United States experience symptoms of a major depressive episode within the course of a typical year [7]. In this case, a major depressive episode is defined as a persistent feeling of sadness or loss of interest associated with changes in sleep, appetite, energy level, concentration, or daily behavior [4]. The Centers for Disease Control and Prevention also reported that 1 out of 8 mothers will experience significant symptoms of postpartum depression after delivery [8]. Shockingly, of those mothers who are affected by postpartum depression, more than 20% will experience suicidal thoughts and 22% will experience severe depression [9]. Unfortunately, although the prevalence rates for mental health disorders, particularly anxiety and depression, are higher during the perinatal period, the treatment rates for these women are consistently lower.

The rate of pregnant and postpartum mothers who receive appropriate mental health care is only around 14% and almost one-half the rate of the general population at 26% [9]. The risk for a woman developing a mood disorder (anxiety or depression) does not decrease after her child-bearing years. In fact, the perimenopausal transition period is often associated with an increased risk for developing or worsening anxiety and depression. Reported estimates of newly diagnosed depression and anxiety in these women are as high as 30% [10]. However, despite this high level of risk, the rate of routine screening of mood disorders remains comparatively low in this population [11].

Why are rates so low in this population? It is highly unlikely that providers are unconcerned with the mental well-being of their patients. Research indicates that providers may not feel confident in their ability to adequately treat

Table 1
Description of unique factors affecting women's mental health

PMS: Premenstrual syndrome:	At least 1 significant affective and 1 significant somatic symptom that cause dysfunction or interfere with normal activities and are cyclical, occurring during the second half of the menstrual cycle, beginning in the 5 d before menses for at least the past 3 cycles. Typically relieved within 4 d of menses and do not recur until cycle day 13 [22].
PMDD: Premenstrual dysphoric disorder	A more severe form of PMS with significant mood symptoms, which may include mood lability, anxiety, depressed mood, anxiety, tension, irritability [4].
Perimenopause	The years in a women's 30s and 40s leading up to menopause. Hormone levels fluctuate, the menstrual cycle changes and may be irregular. Women may experience vasomotor symptoms such as hot flashes, insomnia, and urogenital changes [22].

depression in this age group, have insufficient knowledge, or do not have time during clinical visits for the assessment of behavioral health needs and subsequent referrals [12]. One of the largest considerations to treating psychiatric disorders in women's health are concerns around the teratogenic effects of psychotropic medication before and during pregnancy and through the postdelivery and breast-feeding periods [13]. Although this concern is legitimate, it should be balanced with equally valid concerns for not treating mood disorders in this population. As an example, Grigoriadis and colleagues [14] found that perinatal anxiety is associated with increased risks for preterm birth, lower birth weight, small for gestational age, and smaller head circumference. In many practices across the nation, implementing a system of integrated behavioral health into the practice or an organization has proven to be an effective and practical option for both improving patient outcomes and increasing non–mental health providers confidence in treating mental health conditions, particularly in the management of anxiety and depression [15].

DESCRIPTION OF ONE WOMEN'S HEALTH PRACTICE
The practice presented in this article is a women's health practice that provides comprehensive health care for adolescent and adult women, primary care for women, and low to moderate risk obstetric care. It consists of 30 advanced practice nurses including 23 certified nurse–midwives (CNM) and 7 nurse practitioners (NP), which includes family NPs, women's health NPs, and adult gerontology primary care NPs who provide care to the patient population. This practice is also a teaching facility for the Vanderbilt University School of Nursing, where patients may see numerous providers and students over time. The model of care in this practice focuses on evidence-based, patient-centered care. For calendar year 2020, this practice cared for 2085 patients. Of these patients, 403 (19.3%) had a mental health diagnosis, excluding substance use disorder. Owing to the intimate nature of care provided by this practice, as well as the various providers a patient might see, a standardized method of assessing patients for behavioral health concerns was needed. Research has shown that CoCMs can be effective in obstetrics and gynecology clinics that provide women's health care [16]. It was determined that expanding the behavioral health integration (BHI) model that had been used in primary care practices had the potential to benefit the patient population and providers in a women's health practice.

WHAT IS BEHAVIORAL HEALTH INTEGRATION?
BHI involves incorporating behavioral health services into the health care setting to allow providers to have access to support in addressing their patients' behavioral health needs. The goals of BHI include increased provider comfort with addressing behavioral health needs and an increased availability of behavioral health services for patients. BHI can be in the form of coordinated care with direct referral pathways and consultation, colocated care where providers from behavioral health disciplines share a site and have occasional

communication with the health care providers, or integrated care where behavioral health professionals are incorporated as part of the collaborative treatment team with joint treatment planning [17]. Although there are a variety of BHI models to choose from, they all revolve around a patient-centered and team-based approach to care delivery.

The Advancing Integrated Mental Health Solutions model, more widely known as, the CoCM, was developed by the University of Washington Department of Psychiatry, and it has been implemented in more than 1000 clinics across the United States and abroad [18]. The CoCM revolves around 5 basic principles: (1) patient-centered care, (2) population-based care, (3) measurement-based treat-to-target using evidence-based tools, (4) evidence-based care, and (5) accountable care (Table 2) [18]. The women's health practice decided to implement the widely accepted CoCM and adapt this model, methods, and tools to fit into a nurse-managed women's health setting. The experience of this practice can serve as an example of how behavioral health can be integrated into a women's health practice for those looking to do the same.

INTEGRATION PROCESS AT ONE WOMEN'S HEALTH PRACTICE
A few minor adaptations were required in the CoCM model to accommodate the clinic's advanced nursing foundation. These adaptions included the use of psychiatric mental health NP in place of psychiatrists, the use of licensed social workers (SW) in place of behavioral health coordinators, and the use of the model in a midwifery practice (limited amount of evidence of use in this specialty). Otherwise, the model was implemented as designed. Before the implementation of the CoCM, the primary barriers to mental health care included a low rate of screening and detection of mental health issues, provider comfort

Table 2
Core principles of collaborative care with description

Core Principle	Description
Patient-centered care	Primary care (or other medical) providers and behavioral health providers collaborate to create joint plans of care that take patient goals into consideration
Population-based care	Patients are tracked through a registry shared among team members to track patient improvement
Measurement-based treatment to target	Plans of care include goals and clinical outcomes that can be measured through evidence-based methods. Treatments are actively changed if patients are not improving as expected until the clinical goals are achieved
Evidence-based care	Treatments offered to patients are supported by research evidence that shows they are effective in treating target condition
Accountable care	Providers are accountable for quality of care and clinical outcomes

Adapted from Advanced Integrated Mental Health Systems (AIMS) Center (2019). Program Overview. Retrieved from https://aims.uw.edu/collaborative-care/principles-collaborative-care. Accessed November 2021; with permission.

with treating mental health, delays in patients receiving counseling services, and patients lost in transition to specialty mental health services [19].

A program was developed specific to this practice to create an integrated behavioral health team. This program is designed around SWs acting in the behavioral health coordinator role in a women's health practice. Referrals are received from providers, including CNMs and NPs primarily, who then coordinate care with the SW and psychiatric mental health NP to determine joint treatment plans for each patient. This program has established champion providers in the practice to work directly with the SW to coordinate continuity of patient care and patient follow-up. In this program, a provider identifies a patient with a behavioral health concern using the intake screening process. Providers then use clinical judgment regarding starting medication therapies for patients or consulting with the psychiatric mental health NPs if needed. If behavioral intervention or close follow-up while titrating medications to therapeutic levels is needed, then a referral is placed to the SW for an intake visit. The SW then identifies patient needs through the process and determines a treatment plan with brief behavioral interventions or referral to outside therapies as needed. The SW follows up at regular intervals with the patient, usually beginning with weekly or biweekly visits until established goals are met. Patient tracking is completed using the intake screening and working to reach target goals. Once goals have been met, the SW creates a prevention plan to identify tools and strategies that were successful and how to continue to use these tools if symptoms arise in the future. Patients then return to a typical follow-up care plan with the provider.

Because the prevalence of mood disorders and other behavioral health concerns is high among patients in primary care and women's health settings, universal screening can be beneficial in detecting and addressing these concerns [2]. In this practice, it was determined that using universal screening strategies for anxiety, depression, and suicidality would meet the goal of early identification of behavioral health needs. It is important to use valid and reliable screening tools to identify depression, anxiety, and suicidality concerns for the patient population. This practice chose to use the Patient Health Questionnaire, the Generalized Anxiety Disorder Scale (GAD-7), the Edinburgh Postnatal Depression Scale (EPDS), and the Columbia Suicide Severity Rating Scare as described in Table 3. Patients receive the Patient Health Questionnaire-9 and GAD-7 at every visit with the NPs or SW; patients receive the EPDS and GAD-7 at regular intervals during their pregnancy or postpartum period visits with the CNMs. The American College of Obstetrics and Gynecology recommends screening for postpartum depression and anxiety at a comprehensive postpartum visit, which this practice performs at 6 weeks. This practice also screens all obstetric patients with an EPDS at their first obstetric visit during a pregnancy. Using universal screening allows for the tracking of anxiety and depression symptoms at regular intervals, which is especially important for those who are being treated for mood disorders by providers in the clinical setting.

Table 3
Screening tools used with description and target goals

Screening Tools/ Questionnaires	Tool Description	Target Goals
Patient Health Questionnaire 9- Item (PHQ-9)	9-item tool to detect depressive symptomatology [23]	50% decrease or score of <5
Generalized Anxiety Disorder 7- Item (GAD-7)	7-item tool to detect anxiety symptomatology [23]	50% decrease or score of <10
Columbia-Suicide Severity Rating Scale (C-SSRS)	2-question tool for screening suicidality with extensive severity scale for positive screen [23]	First 2 questions at each encounter. If YES to EITHER question, the full severity scale is initiated. (Note: The Ask Suicide-Screening Questionnaire [ASQ] is preferred if patient is a child or adolescent)
Edinburgh Postnatal Depression Scale (EPDS)	10-question tool to detect perinatal depression and anxiety [24]	50% decrease or score of <10

Measurement-based care that uses this method of tracking has proven to be a more effective way of providing care than standard care. Research has identified that using measurement-based care can decrease the amount of time it takes for a patient to respond to treatment and achieve remission from symptoms [20]. For the BHI program in this practice, measurement-based goals were identified using the screening tools to track patient progress over time. Table 3 identifies the tools and targets goals used is this practice.

DESCRIPTIVE IMPACT OF INTEGRATION IMPLEMENTATION

In 2019, this women's health practice cared for 1283 unique patients and 2085 unique patients in 2020. Of these patients, 17.9% of patients (n = 230) in 2019 and 19.3% of patients (n = 403) in 2020 had an identified mental health diagnosis excluding substance abuse. Ninety-eight percent of encounters with the NPs were screened for depression (Patient Health Questionnaire-9 or EPDS) and anxiety (GAD-7). Two hundred forty patients screened positive for depression or anxiety and could be treated appropriately through the BHI program. Through the treat-to-target and care management components of the model, a total of 101 patients engaged in care with the BHI program and the SW had an average case load of between 35 and 40 patients. Of the 101 patients, 69 graduated (stable with a PQH-9 of <5 or had a 50% decrease), 2 remain active in the program, and only 22 were lost to follow-up or care owing to the inability to connect with the patient. Patient satisfaction has been a focus of this program and, of the patients who have engaged in BHI, 91% reported to be very or extremely satisfied with their care. Patients also reported having felt heard by their provider, satisfied their goals were met in treatment, and equipped upon graduating from the program to address these symptoms in the future [21].

IMPLICATIONS FOR PRACTICE

The adapted CoCM has been highly successful. In this program, patients experienced greater satisfaction with care, a greater likelihood of reaching therapeutic range dosing of medication, and a greater likelihood of a 50% decrease in depression symptoms. Providers identified they felt supported and had increased comfort in treating depression and anxiety. The ability of providers to easily collaborate with the behavioral health team allowed for the creation of cohesive treatment plans and retention of patients who may otherwise be lost to follow-up during the transition to specialty care.

Although primary care NPs are established gatekeepers for their patients where routine screening can provide the identification of behavioral health needs, they face barriers to appropriately treating behavioral health within a primary care setting. Treating behavioral health for women has its own set of specific challenges. In this primary care and women's health practice, barriers to care surrounding pregnancy and the postpartum period, which extended far past the traditional last visit at 6 weeks postpartum, were identified. This practice found a solution by integrating behavioral health into the women's health setting. The implications of BHI are far reaching, but for the purposes of this article, the focus is on the implications for advanced practice nurses, patients, and clinics attempting to provide integrated behavioral health services.

Providers have increased comfort in treating mental health when intimately collaborating with behavioral health professionals. At this practice, this collaboration reaches beyond patients actively enrolled in the BHI program, with providers reporting increased comfort in treating behavioral health needs for traditional patients as well. Providers reported feeling supported and enjoyed the collaboration with behavioral health professionals. They felt better able to practice to the full extent of their scope with regard to mental health services. They felt more confident choosing and starting medications and titrating those medications to therapeutic range dosing. In addition, providers felt more confident broaching difficult conversations, such as suicidality and crisis risk. A supportive environment coupled with repetition lends itself to confident and competent providers.

This practice found the integration of behavioral health to be a significant patient satisfier. Patients who may otherwise be lost to follow-up care are easily able to access mental health care. As this program demonstrates, the integration of behavioral health improves patient outcomes, with greater numbers of patients reaching therapeutic range dosing and reporting improvement in anxiety and depression symptoms through standardized screening. This clinic was a grant-funded program and behavioral services were provided without charge. Although this is practice likely not feasible at most clinics, the authors feel the ease of access, integrated specialized services, and confidence their primary provider has in the behavioral health team is significant enough for patient engagement in an integrated program without grant funding.

This clinic was able to identify areas in which the integration process could be improved and could benefit clinics wishing to implement a similar program. Widely disseminating knowledge of the program to the entire clinic was essential for a cohesive understanding of services and limitations of the BHI program. This process allowed providers to easily identify who was appropriate for care within a BHI program. The authors found that a consistent and simple referral process into the program was essential for expedient scheduling of patients, as well as weeding out inappropriate referrals. Practices looking to implement BHI programs may consider creating a standardized form for use in electronic and paper charting that includes current symptoms, the reason for referral to the BHI program, behavioral health history, comorbidities, current pregnancy or lactation status, and any other pertinent information.

In this clinic, the referral form was sent directly to the SWs, who schedule their own patients. This form also served as a summary for any provider looking within the chart. The clinic initially encountered confusion with scheduling for the correct provider for each visit (NP or CNM vs SW). Patients may only verbalize to scheduling staff they are requesting follow-up for a mood disorder. This can be particularly problematic if interprofessional integration is novel to the practice or the SW role feels unfamiliar to support staff. Scheduling confusion can be mitigated through simple teaching of scheduling practices and the role and scope of the SW, as well as reference guides for scheduling staff. Practices looking to implement BHI programs may find it more straightforward for the SW to schedule their own patients for counseling. The authors found it important to have a standardized interval for scheduled visits with the prescribing provider. In this practice, a good interval for best care is 1 scheduled visit with a prescribing provider for every 4 counseling visits with the SW. Patients may otherwise believe that any needed medication adjustments can occur at counseling visits. This practice allowed for the most complete care of the patient and aided in reaching therapeutic range dosing most efficiently.

When considering scheduling, this practice found these visits were typically appropriate for telehealth with patients completing routine screeners electronically before the start of the telehealth visit. In particular, telehealth visits are a point of satisfaction for newly postpartum mothers. Finally, owing to grant funding and the novelty of this program, the measured outcomes largely focused on clinical impacts. A potential billing implication was increased revenue to the practice simply through increased patient volume. Further work and research may be needed to bridge the clinical and financial impacts of this program.

SUMMARY

In the United States today, women across the nation are experiencing a disparity in mental health care. This issue is due to a myriad of reasons, but those reasons can be summarized into 2 categories. First, in many health care settings, there is a lack of standardized and universal screening to detect even basic mental health conditions, such as anxiety and depressive disorders. Second, many non–mental health providers, including those specializing in women's health, lack the confidence and support to address mental health concerns beyond even the mildest manifestations of the conditions. The intimate collaboration with a BHI team can decrease the number of patients lost to follow-up and falling through the cracks. Although a busy provider does not have the time to routinely reach out to at-risk patients, in integrated behavioral health, a designated SW reaches out to patients at regular intervals to close the gaps in contact between the patient and the clinic. Furthermore, providers are able to care for patients who otherwise may not seek care outside of their established clinic owing to comfort or resources. For those wishing to grow their practice, this method is an excellent way to increase patient retention. With the expansion of primary care services to include addressing mental health needs, patients remain in primary care services who might otherwise transfer to specialty psychiatric care. For those patients with mental health needs with a severity beyond what a primary care or women's health practice can offer, an integrated service can serve as a bridge to specialty care.

Finally, BHI programs are a provider satisfier. Providers report satisfaction with the ease of gaining behavioral health services for patients, feeling supported in care of mental health, and enjoy collaborating with behavioral health providers to form a cohesive treatment plan for optimal patient care. As evidenced by the successful implementation and early positive outcomes of this women's health practice, integrated behavioral health may be a viable solution to mitigate mental health disparity.

Disclosure
Partial funding for this behavioral health integration program was provided by the Health Resources and Services Administration. The authors have no other funding sources to disclose. The authors have no commercial or financial conflict of interest to disclose.

References
[1] National Alliance on Mental Illness. Mental health by the numbers. 2021. Available at: https://www.nami.org/mhstats November 2021.

[2] Trivedi MH, Jha MK, Kahalnik F, et al. VitalSign: a primary care first (PCP-First) model for universal screening and measurement-based care for depression. Pharmaceuticals (Basel) 2019;12(2):71.

[3] Wakida EK, Talib ZM, Akena D, et al. Barriers and facilitators to the integration of mental health services into primary health care: a systematic review. Syst Rev 2018;7:211.

[4] American Psychiatric Association. Diagnostic and statistical manual of mental disorders. 5th edition. American Psychiatric Association; 2013.

[5] The Carter Center. Mental illness will cost the world $16 USD trillion by 2030. Psychiatric Times; 2018 35(11).

[6] Depression in women: understanding the gender gap Mayo Clinic. Available at: https://www.mayoclinic.org/diseases-conditions/depression/in-depth/depression/art-20047725 November 2021.

[7] Zhou J, Ko JY, Haight SC, et al. Treatment of substance use disorders among women of reproductive age by depression and anxiety disorder status, 2008-2014. J Womens Health (Larchmt) 2019;28(8):1068–76.

[8] Depression among women Center for Disease Control. Available at: https://www.cdc.gov/reproductivehealth/depression/index.htm November 2021.

[9] Wisner KL, Sit DK, McShea MC, et al. Onset timing, thoughts of self-harm, and diagnoses in postpartum women with screen-positive depression findings. JAMA Psychiatry 2013;70(5): 490–8.

[10] Cohen LS, Soares CN, Vitonis AF, et al. Risk for new onset of depression during the menopausal transition: the Harvard study of moods and cycles. Arch Gen Psychiatry 2006;63(4): 385–90.

[11] Raglan GB, Schulkin J, Juliano LM, et al. Obstetrician-gynecologists' screening and management of depression during perimenopause. Menopause 2020;27(4):393–7.

[12] Freeman MP. Perinatal depression: recommendations for prevention and the challenges of implementation. J Am Med Assoc 2019;321(6):550–2.

[13] Massachusetts's General Hospital Center for Women's Mental Health (MGHCWMH). Postpartum Psychiatric Disorders. 2019. Available at: https://womensmentalhealth.org/specialty-clinics/postpartum-psychiatric-disorders/ November 2021.

[14] Grigoriadis S, Graves L, Peer M, et al. Maternal anxiety during pregnancy and the association with adverse perinatal outcomes: systematic review and meta-analysis. J Clin Psychiatry 2018;79(5):17r12011.

[15] LaRocco-Cockburn A, Reed SD, Melville J, et al. Improving depression treatment for women: integrating a collaborative care depression intervention into OB-GYN care. Contemp Clin Trials 2013;36(2):362–70 [Erratum appears in Contemp Clin Trials 2014;37(1):166].

[16] Melville JL, Reed SD, Russo J, et al. Improving care for depression in obstetrics and gynecology: a randomized controlled trial. Obstet Gynecol 2014;123(6):1237–46.

[17] Gerrity M. Milbank Memorial Fund. 2016. Available at:https://www.milbank.org/wp-content/uploads/2016/05/Evolving-Models-of-BHI.pdf. November 2021.

[18] Advanced Integrated Mental Health Systems (AIMS) Center. Program Overview. 2019. Available at: https://aims.uw.edu/collaborative-care/principles-collaborative-care November 2021.

[19] Coombs NC, Meriwether WE, Caringi J, et al. Barriers to healthcare access among U.S. adults with mental health challenges: a population-based study. SSM Popul Health 2021;15:100847.

[20] Guo T, Xiang YT, Xiao L, et al. Measurement-based care versus standard care for major depression: a randomized controlled trial with blind raters. Am J Psychiatry 2015;172(10):1004–13.

[21] The Melrose Clinic, 2021. Internal quality improvement data for 2019-2021.

[22] Hofmeister S, Bodden S. Premenstrual syndrome and premenstrual dysphoric disorder. Am Fam Physician 2016;94(3):236–40. Available at: https://www.acog.org/womens-health/faqs, November 2021.

[23] Ketel C, Hedges JP, Smith JP, et al. Suicide detection and treatment in a nurse-led, interprofessional primary care practice. Nurse Pract 2021;46(4):33–40.

[24] Thombs BD, Benedetti A, Kloda LA, et al. Diagnostic accuracy of the Edinburgh Postnatal Depression Scale (EPDS) for detecting major depression in pregnant and postnatal women: protocol for a systematic review and individual patient data meta- analyses. BMJ Open 2015;5:e009742.

The Well-Woman Visit
Adolescence Through End-of-Life

Beth A. Ammerman, DNP, FNP-BC*,
Heather M. Jones, DNP, AGPCNP-C,
Jennifer C. Riske, BSN, RN, OCN,
Elizabeth K. Kuzma, DNP, FNP-BC

Department of Health Behavior and Biological Sciences, University of Michigan School of Nursing, 400 N. Ingalls Street, Ann Arbor, MI 48109, USA

Keywords
- Well-woman visit • Lifespan • Adolescent • Older adult • Childbearing
- Prevention • Health promotion

Key points
- The well-woman visit is an important component of health promotion, disease prevention, and early identification and management of health problems for women.
- The well-woman visit includes a comprehensive patient history, physical examination, routine screening for common conditions, immunizations, health counseling, and anticipatory guidance.
- Although there are many common components to the well-woman visit across age groups, there are unique considerations to the visit by age group.
- The purpose of this article is to provide a resource for primary care nurse practitioners for the well-woman visit by age range including adolescents, adults, and older adults.

INTRODUCTION

The well-woman visit (WWV) is an important component of health promotion, disease prevention, and early identification and management of health problems for women beginning in adolescence and continuing through end-of- life (EOL) [1]. Women primarily receive their annual well visits from a primary care

*Corresponding author. 400 North Ingalls Room 3179, Ann Arbor, MI 48109. *E-mail address:* bammerma@umich.edu

https://doi.org/10.1016/j.yfpn.2021.12.005
2589-420X/22/© 2021 Elsevier Inc. All rights reserved.

provider (PCP) or an obstetrics-gynecology specialist [1]. These visits create the ideal occasion for health care providers (HCP) to establish and maintain relationships with patients, counsel them about health maintenance, and decrease risks for specific conditions [1]. The WWV consists of a detailed, comprehensive patient history, which is arguably the most important component of the visit. Components of a physical examination (PE) determined by age and risk factors, routine screening for common conditions or problems based on age, as well as immunization administration are also included [1]. Although there are many common components to the WWV across the age groups, there are unique considerations to the visit by age group. Routine national guidelines for the different components of the WWV evolve over time and vary based on the organization making the recommendation. The purpose of this article is to provide a resource for practicing primary care nurse practitioners (NPs) for the WWV by age range including adolescents (12–21 years), adults (older than 21 through 64 years), and older adults (older than 65 years).

COMMON WELL-WOMAN NEEDS ACROSS AGE GROUPS

WWVs are extremely important and comprise a large part of the role of a PCP, patient counseling, health maintenance and promotion, disease prevention, and risk reduction [1]. Although not all components of a WWV are recommended annually, it is recommended that women access care for WWVs on a yearly basis. The periodicity for specific assessments and screening tests are individualized based on the patient's age and unique risk factors arising from lifestyle, health behaviors, family history, genetics, past medical history, and current health status [1]. However, regardless of patient age and individual risk factors, there are some key components of the WWV that are consistent across age groups, including components of the patient history and PE. The WWV primarily focuses on the patient relationship, patient history, counseling, and shared decision-making and focuses less on the PE.

SUBJECTIVE

In primary care, the WWV is a comprehensive holistic appointment that includes a detailed health history in addition to a broad screening PE that is more complex than just focusing on breast, pelvic, menstrual, and sexual health [1]. The health history is one of the most important components of the WWV, as it provides essential information about an individual's medical and surgical history, family risk factors, and behaviors that affect a woman's overall health, well-being, and risk for future health problems [2]. To obtain the most accurate patient health history an NP can use patient-centered and motivational interviewing techniques to create a strong patient-provider partnership to help patients achieve their optimal health status [3].

THE HEALTH HISTORY

In general, the components of the well-woman patient history are consistent across all ages, yet there are some unique considerations by age group, which will be laid out later in this article. To begin, the key components of any comprehensive health history for all WWVs are presented.

First, the NP can set the stage for the visit by ensuring privacy and confidentiality for all patients. Although many patients are asked to get undressed and ready for an examination before the provider entering the room, it is much more respectful to have the patient remain dressed for the health history because the history portion of a WWV can take a bit of time to complete. The patient will likely feel much more comfortable and relaxed answering questions while they are fully clothed [4]. The NP can then work to establish the patient-provider relationship, which includes treating the patient with respect [5,6]. This relationship can be accomplished by establishing the patient's preferred name and always asking the patient for proper pronunciation of their name [5,6], and this is also a good time to assess the patient's gender identity, sex assigned at birth, preferred pronouns (eg, he/him/his; she/her/hers; they/them/theirs), and sexual orientation, if not already collected on intake forms [7]. This is very important, because if the patient identifies as a transgender man, and still has a uterus and cervix, they should be screened for cervical cancer [8]. If the patient is a transgender woman, they will not need cervical cancer screening [8]. When assessing gender identity and sexual orientation, ask the questions in a straightforward, respectful manner. The more comfortable the NP is and the more the NP normalizes the questions, the more at ease the patient will be [8].

Examples of appropriate questions include the following [9]:

1. "Do you think of yourself as: lesbian, gay, or homosexual, straight or heterosexual, bisexual, something else, don't know?" [9].
2. "What sex were you assigned at birth, such as on an original birth certificate?" [9].
3. "Do you have any concerns or questions about your sexuality, sexual orientation, or sexual desires?" [9].

Sexual and gynecologic history

A comprehensive sexual health history for the WWV includes the 6 Ps (partners, practices, protection from sexually transmitted infections (STIs), past history of STIs, prevention of pregnancy, and pleasure) as listed in Table 1 [10]. Along with the sexual history, a detailed gynecologic and menstrual history are essential components of the WWV [1].

Well-woman gynecologic and menstrual history questions include the following:

- Menses [11]
  - Age of menarche
  - Menstrual cycle length, flow, frequency, and associated symptoms
  - Age of menopause
  - Any postmenopausal bleeding
- Pregnancy history [1]
  - Including any pregnancies, fertility issues, births, abortions (elective, spontaneous, missed), surgeries, current and planned contraception (if indicated), and family planning within the next year.

Table 1
Health history

Health History (Acronym: SMASH FM) [12]	
Surgical	Including obstetric/gynecologic surgeries (eg, cesarean sections)
Medical	Illnesses, fractures, injuries
Allergies	Include the type of allergic reaction
Immunizations	Include all childhood/adult immunizations
Hospitalizations	Injuries, illnesses, childbirths
Family history	Illnesses of biological siblings, parents, grandparents, children
Medications	Prescribed, over-the-counter (OTC), natural, vitamins/supplements, home remedies

Social History (Acronym: FED TACOS) [13]	
• Food/Diet	24-h diet recall; food insecurity
• Exercise	How much, how often, types
• Drugs	Recreational drugs, marijuana, OTC
• Tobacco use	Smoking, chewing, vaping
• Alcohol	Amount, frequency, CAGE questionnaire (C: Cutting Down, A: Annoyance by Criticism, G: Guilty Feeling, E: Eye-openers)
	• https://archives.drugabuse.gov/publications/resource-guide-screening-drug-use-in-general-medical-settings/nida-quick-screen
• Caffeine	Coffee, tea, soda, energy drinks, oral supplements
• Occupation/Living	All women: safe living, workplace or environmental exposures; relationships, relaxation, money/pay bills
• Sexual history	6 Ps: partners, practices, protection from STIs, past STIs, prevention of pregnancy, pleasure
Safety/interpersonal violence Assessment [14]	• Have you ever been hit, kicked, slapped, or otherwise physically hurt by someone close to you?
	• Have you ever been forced to engage in sexual activities that you did not want to?
Full review of systems	• General
	• Integumentary
	• HEENOT, including dental health
	• Cardiovascular
	• Respiratory
	• Abdominal
	• Genitourinary
	• Gynecologic
	• Musculoskeletal
	• Neurologic
	• Chest/breasts
	• Mental health
	• Hematologic
	• Endocrine
Injury prevention/risk reduction behaviors	• Use of helmets, seatbelts, & protective sporting equipment
	• Use of personal protective equipment in jobs
	• Use of facemasks, social distancing, & handwashing/hygiene
Is there anything else you would like to discuss today?	

Data from Bickley LS. Bates' Guide to Physical Examination and History Taking. 12th ed. Wolters Kluwer. 2017.

- ○ Asking "Would you like to become pregnant in the next year?" is clear, to the point, and professional.
- Gynecologic specific symptoms (helps determine what type of examination is indicated) [11].
  - ○ Vaginal discharge, itching, odor, lesions
  - ○ Pain with sexual activity
  - ○ Bleeding with sex, bleeding between cycles

The full components of the health history are listed in Table 1.

OBJECTIVE

A comprehensive annual PE is recommended as part of the WWV for women of all ages. However, not all components of a PE are required at every visit [1]. NPs providing primary care to women can determine whether or not the pelvic and breast examinations are recommended based on the patient's health history, age, and individual risk factors [1]. Currently, unless a woman is being screened for cervical cancer, it is recommended to not perform a pelvic examination on an asymptomatic woman during a routine wellness check-up [15]. If the patient has symptoms, of course a pelvic examination may be necessary. There is no reason to perform a pelvic examination for the routine prescribing of oral contraceptives [16]. If a pelvic and/or breast examination is indicated, an NP can engage in shared decision-making with the patient about whether the examination will be performed [1]. The components of the well-woman PE across all ages are listed in Box 1.

SCREENING

The WWV examination includes several screening assessments, some that are relevant to all women regardless of age and others that are unique to their age and individual risk factors. The screening assessments relevant to women across all ages are listed in Table 2.

HEALTH COUNSELING AND ANTICIPATORY GUIDANCE

There are standard topics that should be included in any patient counseling and anticipatory guidance during an annual WWV regardless of patient age, including those listed as follows [2]:

- Nutritional counseling
- Physical activity counseling
- Smoking cessation counseling (if indicated)
- Alcohol reduction counseling (if indicated)

UNIQUE AGE-BASED CONSIDERATIONS FOR THE WELL-WOMAN VISIT

Aspects of the WWV also include age and developmental specific history, PE screenings, and counseling. In addition to those aspects listed earlier,

Box 1: Physical examination

Physical Examination

This will be dictated by patient history but the following may apply:

Vitals signs (height, weight, BMI, waist circumference, temperature, pulse, respirations, BP)

General

HEENOT

Cardiac

Respiratory

Chest/Breast examination

Abdomen

Neurologic/Mental status

Musculoskeletal

Mental health/Psychological

Gynecologic (if indicated including Pap test or symptomatic)

Vision

Hearing

Abbreviations: BMI, body mass index; BP, blood pressure; HEENOT, head, ears, eyes, nose, oral, and throat examination.

Data from Bickley LS. Bates' Guide to Physical Examination and History Taking.12th ed. Wolters Kluwer. 2017

following are the age-specific aspects to consider in performing well-woman examinations.

ADOLESCENT WOMEN'S HEALTH (12–21 YEARS)

There are several unique components to the adolescent female wellness visit (age 12–21 years). Often adolescent well visits for young women aged 12 to 17 years begin with the parent in the room to help with the health history and be present for the PE [22]. However, it is essential that young women aged 12 to 17 years have the opportunity to speak alone with their HCP, such as an NP; this helps young adolescent women to take more ownership of their health, helps to establish an individual relationship with their HCP, and allows the opportunity to discuss issues young women often do not feel comfortable discussing in front of their parents [23]. Of utmost importance is to explain and review minor consent laws and let them know when you would be legally required to disclose information [23,24]. By explaining rules and laws upfront, a provider clearly communicates to young women what they can discuss in confidentiality; this can create trust and assure transparency between the HCP and the young woman. Young women aged 18 to 21 years are legally able to consent to their own health care, so they do not fall under the minor

Table 2	
Routine well-woman screening from adolescence to end-of-life	
Anxiety Screening [17]	• The Women's Preventive Services Initiative (WPSI) recommends screening for anxiety in women & adolescent girls aged 13 y or older who are not currently diagnosed with anxiety disorders, including pregnant & postpartum women.
	• Optimal screening intervals are unknown, & clinical judgment should be used to determine frequency. When screening suggests the presence of anxiety, further evaluation is necessary to establish the diagnosis & determine appropriate treatment and follow-up (FU).
	• GAD-7: https://adaa.org/sites/default/files/GAD-7_Anxiety-updated_0.pdf
Depression Screening [18,19]	• Age 12 y & older should have annual depression screening
	• PHQ-9 https://www.apa.org/depression-guideline/patient-health-questionnaire.pdf
Social Determinants of Health [20,21]	• Food insecurity: ever eat less than you think you should because there is not enough food
	• Housing instability: are you concerned about your ability to obtain safe secure housing
	• Difficulty with transportation getting to/from work, school, or health care appointments
	• Ability to pay utility bills: ever had utilities shut off due to inability to pay?

consent laws and limits. Unique components to the adolescent health history for adolescent women are outlined in Table 3.

SUBJECTIVE
Objective
There are a few examinations that are unique to the adolescent patient, including an assessment for scoliosis, Tanner staging, and assessing a functional Duck Walk for youth in sports [2]. Screening for scoliosis begins in children at age 10 years and continues through age 18 years for adolescents [26]. An in-office test for scoliosis typically includes the forward bend test, with or without the addition of additional screening mechanisms with a scoliometer measurement or Moiré topography [26]. Tanner staging is an important component of the well adolescent female examination and is the gold standard to evaluate adolescent development of secondary sexual characteristics, for example, breast and pubic hair development [2]. The functional Duck Walk is used for the sports physical and is unique to this age group. It yields information about range of motion, joint stability, balance, flexibility, and agility and to test for meniscus tears [2]. See Table 4 for unique screening recommendations for young women aged 12 to 21 years.

HEALTH COUNSELING AND ANTICIPATORY GUIDANCE
There are standard topics that should be included as part of routine patient counseling and anticipatory guidance during an annual WWV for adolescent

Table 3
Unique health history for women ages 12 to 21 years

Adolescent Risk Assessment	• General Resource Document: https://umhs-adolescenthealth.org/wp-content/uploads/2017/10/adolescent-risk-screening-starter-guide.pdf
	• HEADSS (Home, Education, Activities, Drugs, Sex, Suicide) http://www.bcchildrens.ca/Youth-Health-Clinic-site/Documents/headss20assessment20guide1.pdf
	• Guidelines for Adolescent Preventive Services
	  ○ Age 11–14 y: https://www.uvpediatrics.com/Docs/GAPS11-14Eng.pdf
	  ○ Age 15–21 y: https://www.uvpediatrics.com/Docs/GAPS15-21Eng.pdf
	• Rapid Adolescent Prevention Screening https://possibilitiesforchange.org/raaps/

Bullying [25]	How often do you…
	1. Get picked on by other kids:
	  ☐ Never ☐ Once in a while ☐ Pretty often ☐ Often
	2. Get made fun of:
	  ☐ Never ☐ Once in a while ☐ Pretty often ☐ Often
	3. Get called names by other kids:
	  ☐ Never ☐ Once in a while ☐ Pretty often ☐ Often
	4. Get hit and pushed:
	  ☐ Never ☐ Once in a while ☐ Pretty often ☐ Often

Growth and Development	• Age 12–14 y: https://www.cdc.gov/ncbddd/childdevelopment/positiveparenting/adolescence.html • Age 15–17 y: https://www.cdc.gov/ncbddd/childdevelopment/positiveparenting/adolescence2.html
School Performance	Grade in school/education level, academic performance, extracurricular activities, friends

Table 4
Unique screening for women ages 12 to 21 years

Routine well-woman screening and immunizations ages 12–21 y	
Immunizations	Birth through age 18 y: • https://www.cdc.gov/vaccines/schedules/hcp/imz/child-adolescent.html 19 y & older: • https://www.cdc.gov/vaccines/schedules/hcp/imz/adult.html

STI recommendations for screening [27]	• Chlamydia & gonorrhea:
	  ○ Sexually active women younger than 25 y [27]
	• Human immunodeficiency virus:
	  ○ All women aged 13–64 y (opt-out) [27]
	  ○ Recommended to treat prophylactically with PrEP (pre-exposure prophylaxis medication) if high risk
	• Hepatitis C (HCV):
	  ○ All adults older than 18 y should be screened for hepatitis C except in settings where the HCV positivity is < 0.1% [27]

young women, including those listed earlier, while using motivational interviewing strategies and techniques.

- Risk reduction behaviors [2,28]:
  - https://nahic.ucsf.edu/resource_center/adolescent-guidelines/
  - https://pediatrics.aappublications.org/content/145/3/e20200013
- Safety [28]:
  - Helmet use every time with use of a skateboard, bicycle, scooter, hoverboard, or snowboard
  - Regular and consistent seatbelt use every time in a car, no matter where sitting in the car
  - Not texting and driving or riding in the car with someone who is texting and driving
  - Not drinking and driving or riding in the car with someone who has been drinking alcohol
  - Sun safety: limiting time out in the sun, using sunscreen when out in the sun for prolonged periods of time, wearing clothing and hats as sun protection
- Contraception counseling [28].
- STI prevention counseling [28].
- Fertility awareness counseling [29,30].

WOMEN'S HEALTH (OLDER THAN 21 THROUGH 64 YEARS)
Subjective

Women older than 21 through 64 years require additional preventative health measures included in their well visits. In addition to a detailed health history, women in this age group should be screened for communicable diseases, drug and alcohol misuse, mental health concerns, as well as specific cancer and cardiac screenings [1,2]. Guidelines for any routine screenings outlined are for average-risk individuals and require thoughtful conversation with patients about personal and familial risk factors as outlined in the previous section about the Health History in the Common Well-Woman Needs Across Age Groups (see Table 1). Unique screening recommendations for this age group are outlined in Table 5.

OBJECTIVE
The PE for women older than 21 up to 65 years is guided by the individual history and active problem list and may be similar to the adolescent patient.

Health counseling and anticipatory guidance
There are standard topics that should be included as part of routine patient counseling and anticipatory guidance during an annual WWV for women older than 21 years through the age of 64 years, including those listed as follows, while using motivational interviewing strategies and techniques.

- Preconception and family planning [55]: women older than 21 years through the age of 64 years represent the largest age group for childbearing.

Table 5
Unique health history for women older than 21 up to 65 years

Routine well-woman screening, counseling, and immunizations ages 21–65 y	
Breast cancer screening	• Guidelines vary based on organization (American College of Obstetrics and Gynecology [ACOG], United States Preventive Services Task Force [USPSTF], American Cancer Society [ACS], American College of Radiology [ACR], American Association of Family Physicians [AAFP], American College of Physicians [ACP], International Agency for Research on Cancer [IARC]) • Shared decision-making (SDM) is key between the provider & patient • The Centers for Disease Control and Prevention (CDC) has created a very informative comparison of breast cancer screening national guidelines into one resource for clinicians, which is updated regularly. It is titled Breast Cancer Screening Guidelines for Women: https://www.cdc.gov/cancer/breast/pdf/breast-cancer-screening-guidelines-508.pdf

Cardiovascular disease (CVD) screening: cardiovascular screening is recommended for all women, ages 20 y & older; routine screening for low-risk patients should take place every 5 y [32,33]. The frequency also depends on age, health status, & other comorbidities	Beyond a comprehensive health history, CVD screening includes looking for risk factors:
	• Obesity screening [31]:
	  ○ Height & weight, body mass index (BMI), & waist circumference measurements yearly.
	  ○ Counseling: behavioral interventions (diet & physical activity for weight loss)
	• Hypertension screening/blood pressure [31] reading in office:
	  ○ 18–39-year-olds, every 3–5 y if not at increased risk
	  ○ 18–39-year-olds, annually for those with increased risk
	  ○ 40 y & older, annually
	• Lipid screening recommendations [32,33]:
	  ○ Every 5 y for people age 20 y or older who are at low risk for CVD.
	  ○ More frequently than every 5 y for people with CVD risk factors.
	• Diabetes screening: see later
	• Tobacco cessation [34]: all patients older than 13 y, ask yearly about tobacco use, provide smoking cessation counseling to those who smoke
	• Screening resting or exercise electrocardiogram (ECG) [35]:
	  ○ Low risk: not recommended

(continued on next page)

Table 5 (continued)	
Routine well-woman screening, counseling, and immunizations ages 21–65 y	
	○ Intermediate or high risk: insufficient evidence for recommendation either for or against getting resting or exercise ECG
• Lipid treatment based on CVD estimate [36]:
○ 40–75 y of age: if one or more CVD risk factors present & calculated 10 y risk of a CVD event is = or >10%, consider starting a statin to prevent CVD (ie, dyslipidemia, diabetes, hypertension, or smoking)
○ https://tools.acc.org/ASCVD-Risk-Estimator-Plus/#!/calculate/estimate/
Cervical cancer screening [37,38]	• Guidelines exist regardless of human papilloma virus (HPV) vaccine status
• Guidelines vary based on the organization
• USPSTF guidelines are supported by ACOG [37]:
○ Begin screening at age 21 y. If a woman has not had sex by age 21 y, may postpone if no risk factors
○ 21–29 y of age: pap test alone every 3 y, with first Pap test at age 21 y
○ 30–65 y of age Pap recommendations are
▪ Pap only every 3 y, or
▪ Pap + hrHPV cotesting every 5 y, or
▪ hrHPV testing alone every 5 y
○ >65 y with normal risk: no cervical screening needed if they have had adequate screening (had normal screens in the past 10 y with cytology, cotest, or HPV screen alone at recommended intervals)
• ACS 2020 guidelines recommend [38]:
○ Begin screening at age 25 y, not 21 y
○ 25–65 y
▪ HPV test alone every 5 y (preferred)
▪ HPV/Pap cotest every 5 y (acceptable)
▪ Pap test alone every 3 y (acceptable)
○ Older than 65 y: no screening as long as series of prior tests were normal
• American Society for Colposcopy and Cervical Pathology (ASCCP) supports both the USPSTF & the new ACS guidelines [37]
• And everyone seems to agree on the following [37]:
○ Women who had hysterectomy for noncancerous reasons: no screening recommended

(continued on next page)

Table 5
(continued)

Routine well-woman screening, counseling, and immunizations ages 21–65 y

	○ If a woman has had a supracervical hyster-ectomy (partial hysterectomy) & still has a cervix, she should continue with current cervical screening guidelines for her age
	○ Women may require more frequent cervical screening based on risk factors
	○ Special considerations exist for women with the following conditions:
	  ▪ Had in utero exposure to diethylstilbestrol (DES)
	  ▪ Have a compromised immune system (human immunodeficiency virus [HIV], long-term steroid use)
	  ▪ Previously had gynecologic cancer, including treatment of a high-grade precancerous lesion or cervical cancer

Colorectal cancer screening [39]	• Routine screening should begin at age 45 or 50 y, depending on the guideline used & stop at 75 years old for most women
	• the age 45 y is a relatively new recommendation, there are some third-party payers who will currently only pay for routine screening after age 50 y, but expect that to change as the newer guidelines become more widely accepted
	• Acceptable forms of screening include:
	  ○ Annual fecal immunochemical test (FIT) or high-sensitivity guaiac-based fecal occult blood test (HSgFOBT)
	  ○ DNA-FIT (FIT test & another test that detects altered DNA in the stool) every 1–3 y
	  ○ Computerized tomography (CT) colonography every 5 y
	  ○ Flexible sigmoidoscopy every 5 y
	  ○ Flexible sigmoidoscopy plus annual FIT
	  ○ Colonoscopy every 10 y
	**A digital rectal examination with occult blood testing performed in the office is not sufficient testing & is not recommended.*
	• If a young woman has a first-degree relative with a history of colorectal cancer, her screening should begin 10 y before the age at which the family member was diagnosed

Diabetes screening [40–43]	USPSTF recommendations for prediabetes/type 2 diabetes mellitus (DM) screening [40]: • 35–70 y of age with overweight or obese: every 3 y

(continued on next page)

Table 5
(*continued*)

Routine well-woman screening, counseling, and immunizations ages 21–65 y

	• Pregnancy 24 wk gestation: screen for gestational diabetes [41]
	Women's Preventive Services Initiative (WPSI) [42]:
	• ≥ 13 y with previous gestational diabetes (GD): every 3 y for at least 10 y after pregnancy
	American Diabetes Association (ADA) [43]:
	• Begin at 45 y for low risk & repeat every 3 y
	• Women with history of GD: every 3 y for life
	Acceptable glucose screenings include [43]:
	• Fasting plasma glucose
	○ 100–125 is consistent with prediabetes
	○ >126 indicates greater risk of type 2 DM
	• Hemoglobin A1c (HbA1c) level
	○ 5.7%–6.4% is consistent with prediabetes
	○ >6.5% is consistent with type 2 DM
	• Oral glucose tolerance test (OGTT):
	○ 2-h postload glucose levels of 140–199 mg/dL (7.77–11.04 mmol/L) are consistent with prediabetes
	○ 2-h postload glucose level of 200 mg/dL (11.1 mmol/L)
Immunizations	https://www.cdc.gov/vaccines/schedules/hcp/imz/adult.html
Lung cancer screening [44]	low-dose CT: annual screening for lung cancer with low-dose computed tomography (LDCT) screening in patients who are
	• 55–80 years old
	• 30 pack-year history of smoking
	• Current smokers or have quit within the past 15 y
	• Screening should cease after 15 y postquitting or if the woman has a serious illness that would limit her ability to have curative lung surgery
Osteoporosis screening [45–47]	• Not routine until age 65 y
	• Although a baseline bone density imaging screening is routinely performed after age 65 y, those at high risk may have this done at a younger age
	• Screening tools used to assess risk in those younger than 65 y. Some common ones include
	○ Simple Calculated Osteoporosis Risk Estimation (SCORE; https://www.medicalalgorithms.com/simplified-calculated-osteoporosis-risk-estimation-tool)

(*continued on next page*)

Table 5
(continued)

Routine well-woman screening, counseling, and immunizations ages 21–65 y	
	○ Fracture Risk Assessment (FRAX) tool (https://www.sheffield.ac.uk/FRAX/) Risk factors for osteoporotic fractures at younger than 65 y include [46,47]: • Hip fracture in a parent • Fracture > age 45 y • Heavy smoking • Alcohol consumption of >3 drinks/d • BMI < 22 • Long-term use of glucocorticosteroids >3 mo (>5 mg prednisolone daily) If the screening tool is positive, the typical test that is ordered [45–47]: • Dual-energy X-ray absorptiometry (DEXA) scan

STI recommendations for screening	• Chlamydia & gonorrhea:
	  ○ Sexually active women younger than 25 y [27]
	  ○ Sexually active women older than 25 y with risk factors:
	    ▪ those who have a new sex partner
	    ▪ >1 sex partner or their partner has >1 partner
	    ▪ A sex partner who has an STI [27]
	• HIV:
	  ○ All women aged 13–64 y (opt-out) [27]
	  ○ Recommended to treat prophylactically with PREP if high risk [48]
	• Hepatitis C (HCV):
	  ○ All adults older than 18 y should be screened for hepatitis C except in settings where the HCV positivity is < 0.1% [27]

Skin cancer screening [49–51]	Few professional organizations outline clinical guidelines or recommendations for screening for skin cancer, including USPSTF, AAFP, ACS, American Academy of Dermatology (AADA), and the Skin Cancer Foundation [49]
	• USPSTF [50]:
	  ○ No recommendation for screening due to insufficient data to support for or against screening for skin cancer
	  ○ USPSTF recommendation to counsel: counsel fair-skinned young adults, adolescents, children, & parents of young children about minimizing exposure to ultraviolet radiation to reduce risk of skin cancer (ages 6 mo to 24 y)
	• Proposed skin cancer screening guidelines from *Melanoma Management* Journal [49]:

(continued on next page)

Table 5 (continued)	
Routine well-woman screening, counseling, and immunizations ages 21–65 y	
	○ Screen women age 35–75 y annually with one or more risk factors with a total body skin examination of the entire surface of the skin: ■ Risk factors include personal history of melanoma, actinic keratosis, keratinocyte carcinoma, or immunocompromised; family history of melanoma; physical characteristics of fair skin, light hair (red or blonde), many freckles, severe sun damaged skin, 2 or more atypical nevi, and/or >40 total nevi; history of indoor tanning &/or peeling or blistering sunburns • National Cancer Institute: ○ Screening for skin cancer may include examination by both the patient & the HCP [51]
Urinary incontinence screening	Screen women of all ages and postpartum women annually [52,53] • Questionnaire for Urinary Incontinence (QUID) is a validated tool that is easy to use: https://www.sclhealth.org/-/media/files/shared/patients-visitors/questionnaire-for-urinary-incontinence-diagnosis.pdf [54]

Therefore, issues of fertility, family planning, infertility, menstrual health, and menopause all hallmark the care of the adult woman older than 21 through 64 years.

- During the annual WWV, it is essential to collect a detailed menstrual history for women in this age group [55]. A comprehensive menstrual history includes assessment of age of menarche, last menstrual period, flow/volume, dysmenorrhea, regularity of menses, age of onset of menopause, and any postmenopausal bleeding. Family planning, fertility, and preconception counseling includes an assessment of the history of contraception use, pregnancy and birth history, history of any abortions (spontaneous, elected, missed), and any complications with pregnancies or births.
- Folic acid supplementation recommendations [55] 400 to 800 µg daily for prevention of spinal cord deformities in women planning pregnancy.

WOMEN'S HEALTH (AGE 65 YEARS AND OLDER)
Subjective
Important considerations when performing the patient history of an older adult woman include any problems with hearing loss, visual impairment, and cognition to ensure appropriate communication [56]. There are several specific components to the older adult WWV (age 65 years and older), much that are

Table 6
Unique screening for women ages 65 years and older

Routine well-woman screening and immunizations ages 65+	
Blood pressure screening	Blood pressure in older woman should be checked at least once a year, more often in the presence of diabetes, heart disease, kidney problems, or other medical conditions or known hypertension [57].
Breast cancer screening	Breast cancer screenings continue into this age group & the specific recommendations for the woman older than 65 y include: • A clinical breast examination may be done every 1–2 y, but recommendations vary on this [58]. • Mammograms are recommended in older women up to age 75 y every 1–2 y depending on risk factors [58]. • Mammography can continue in older women in good health using SDM considering quality of life & longevity [1,58].
Cervical cancer screening	Recommendation is to stop cervical cancer screening in women with an intact cervix after age 65 y who [37,38]: • Do not have a history of cancer or precancer, AND • Have had (3) negative cytology tests in the last 10 y OR • (2) consecutive normal cytology with HPV contesting in the last 10 y & the most recent test was within 5 y. OR • Have no other risk factors Still need Pap tests if [57]: • Exposed to diethylstilbestrol (DES) before birth • Have a weak immune system • HIV positive • History of cervical cancer • Inadequate testing before age 65 y • Have a new sexual partner OR are current or previous smokers with a life expectancy of >10 y generally should continue to be screened for cervical cancer
Cognitive assessment	MMSE only in those with cognitive complaints, either reported by the patient or caregiver or observed by a clinician [57] https://www.dementiacarecentral.com/mini-mental-state-exam/

Colorectal cancer screening	• Routine screening should begin at 45 or 50 y, depending on the guideline used & stop at 75 y for most women [39].
	• Because age 45 y is a relatively new recommendation, there are some third-party payers who will currently only pay for routine screening after age 50 y but expect that to change as the newer guidelines become more widely accepted [39].
	• Acceptable forms of screening include [39]:
	  ○ Annual fecal immunochemical test (FIT) or high-sensitivity guaiac-based fecal occult blood test (HSgFOBT)
	  ○ DNA-FIT every 1–3 y;
	  ○ Computerized tomography colonography every 5 y
	  ○ Flexible sigmoidoscopy every 5 y
	  ○ Flexible sigmoidoscopy plus annual FIT
	  ○ Colonoscopy every 10 y
	**A digital rectal examination with occult blood testing performed in the office is not sufficient testing & is not recommended. [39]

(continued on next page)

Table 6 *(continued)*	
Routine well-woman screening and immunizations ages 65+	
	Colorectal cancer screenings continue into this age group & the specific recommendations for the woman older than 65 y include [59]:
	• 65–75 y of age: the older woman should have colorectal cancer screening at regular intervals until age 75 y
	• Women > 75 y: the continuation of colorectal cancer screening should be discussed using SDM, quality of life, & life expectancy.
	• Colorectal cancer screening tests should be avoided on asymptomatic women who:
	○ Have a life expectancy of <10 y
	○ No family or personal history of colorectal cancer
Diabetes screening	In the absence of diabetes, prediabetes, obesity, or other risk factors, screening for diabetes should occur at least every 3 y [57].
Driving safety assessment	https://www.ncbi.nlm.nih.gov/pmc/articles/PMC4872183/
ECG	Once per lifetime screening for Welcome to Medicare [60]
Fall risk assessment	Assessment for risk for falls should be completed at least once a year including frequency of falling & difficulties in gait or balance [61]. https://www.cdc.gov/steadi/pdf/TUG_test-print.pdf
Functional and home safety assessment	Home safety and functional screening assessments including basic activities of daily living (BADLS) and instrumental activities of daily living (IADLS) should be performed whenever there is a change in functional status [61] https://www.ncbi.nlm.nih.gov/pmc/articles/PMC5928588/ https://www.cdc.gov/homeandrecreationalsafety/pubs/english/booklet_eng_desktop-a.pdf
Hearing screening	USPSTF concluded there was insufficient evidence to determine screening guidelines in asymptomatic adults; however, it is suggested to screen those with functional decline or cognitive problems, which can be easily done in the primary care office with the Whispered Voice Test [56,57].
Hyperlipidemia screening	If cholesterol is normal, women should have it rechecked at least every 5 y. In the presence of hyperlipidemia, diabetes, heart disease, kidney disease, or other conditions it will need to be checked more often [57].
Immunizations	https://www.cdc.gov/vaccines/schedules/hcp/imz/adult.html
Osteoporosis screening [45–47]	• Not routine until age 65 y
	• Although a baseline bone density imaging screening is routinely performed after age 65 y, those at high risk may have this done at a younger age
	• Screening tools used to assess risk in those younger than 65 y. Some common ones include:
	○ Simple Calculated Osteoporosis Risk Estimation (SCORE; https://www.medicalalgorithms.com/simplified-calculated-osteoporosis-risk-estimation-tool),

(continued on next page)

Table 6 (continued)	
Routine well-woman screening and immunizations ages 65+	
	o Fracture Risk Assessment (FRAX) tool (https://www.sheffield.ac.uk/FRAX/) Risk factors for osteoporotic fractures younger than 65 y include [46,47]: • Hip fracture in a parent • Fracture > age 45 y • Heavy smoking • Alcohol consumption of >3 drinks/d • BMI < 22 • Long-term use glucocorticosteroids > 3 mo (>5 mg prednisolone daily) If the screening tool is positive, the typical test that is ordered [45–47]: • Dual-energy X-ray absorptiometry (DEXA) scan All women starting at age 65 y should have a DEXA scan [57]. Further follow-up DEXA scans are recommended as follows [57]: • Adults with low bone mass (T-score: −2.00 to −2.49) at risk for ongoing bone loss, every 2 y as long as the risk factor persists • Women aged 65 y or older at baseline screening with low bone mass (T-score: −1.50 to −1.99) at any site & no risk factors, follow-up in 3–5 y • Women aged 65 y or older at baseline screening with normal or slightly low bone mass (T-score: −1.01 to −1.49) & no risk factors for accelerated bone loss, a follow-up DEXA in 10–15 y
Vision screening	Snellen eye chart examination in the office can be performed; however, there is no clear indication to perform regularly scheduled screenings among otherwise asymptomatic, average-risk older adults. Screening should be considered in those with functional impairment, falls, or cognitive decline [56,57].

associated with age-related changes, including the addition of a functional assessment, cognitive assessment with the mini mental status examination (MMSE), home safety assessment, and driving safety, which are outlined in Table 6.

OBJECTIVE

The individual PE for women ages 65 years and older is guided by history and active problem list; this may be similar to the examination for women aged 12 to 64 years. However, extra care should be taken with consideration of the physical capacity and limitations of the older adult woman [56]. Beginning at age 65 years, women also begin their annual Medicare Wellness Visits (MWV), with the "Welcome to Medicare Visit" also known as the "Initial Preventive Physical Examination," followed by the Initial Annual Wellness visit and Subsequent Annual Wellness visits. Information detailing MWV

Table 7
Resources

Organization	Description	Web site
American College of Obstetrics and Gynecology (ACOG): WWV Health Care	National organization that produces practice guidelines for clinicians & educational materials for patients aimed at improving women's health.	https://www.acog.org/topics/well-woman-health-care?utm_source=redirect&utm_medium=web&utm_campaign=otn
ASCCP Risk-Based Evaluation	Pap smear guidelines	https://www.asccp.org/management-guidelines
Bright Futures	National health promotion & prevention initiative to provide clinicians tools for managing well child & adolescent care. Its usability is helpful beyond designated age groups.	https://brightfutures.aap.org/Bright%20Futures%20Documents/BF4_AdolescenceVisits.pdf https://brightfutures.aap.org/materials-and-tools/tool-and-resource-kit/Pages/adolescence-tools.aspx
CDC Immunization Schedules	Links to immunization schedules by age: • Birth–age 18 y • Adults 19 y & up	https://www.cdc.gov/vaccines/schedules/index.html
Choosing Wisely Promoting conversations between patients & clinicians	Initiative to increase dialogue on avoiding unnecessary medical tests, treatments, & procedures.	www.choosingwisely.org
Nurse Practitioner Women's Health WWV Practice Guidelines	Women's health nurse practitioners organization that champions state-of-the-science health care that holistically addresses the unique needs of women across their lifetimes. Free mobile app is designed for clinicians that is a helpful tool for the WWV	https://www.npwh.org/pages/mobile-app
One Key Question	Reproductive Intentions/Pregnancy Desires Assessment	https://powertodecide.org/one-key-question

(continued on next page)

Table 7
(continued)

Organization	Description	Web site
United States Preventive Services Task Force (USPSTF)	National evidence-based recommendations about clinical preventive services.	https://www.uspreventiveservicestaskforce.org/uspstf/ https://www.uspreventiveservicestaskforce.org/apps/
Women's Preventative Services Initiative	Partnership between ACOG & the US Department of Health and Human Services and Health Resources and Services Administration (HRSA) to develop, review, & update recommendations for women's preventive health care services.	https://www.womenspreventivehealth.org/

requirements and optional assessments can be found at https://www.cms.gov/Outreach-and-Education/Medicare-Learning-Network-MLN/MLNProducts/preventive-services/medicare-wellness-visits.html. Unique screening recommendations for this age group are outlined in Table 6.

Health counseling and anticipatory guidance

- Nutrition counseling: the American Geriatric Society recommends serum vitamin D level of 30 to be the minimal goal in older adults. Most experts advise that daily vitamin D intake in older women be 800 IU including at least 1200 mg of calcium either supplemented or in the diet [57].
- Routine weight measurements, nutritional assessments, inquiring about appetite, food security, swallowing ability [57].
- Injury prevention (falls): the American Heart Association/American College of Sports Medicine recommends specific exercises that can help prevent falls in the older woman. These include aerobic activity, muscle strengthening, flexibility, and balance training exercises for adults older than 65 y [62].
- Advance Care Planning: often happens during an optional component during an Annual Wellness Visit; however, conversations can be started at any time [60,63].

SUMMARY

Well-woman care is a critical role of the primary care NP, and this article can serve as a clinical resource for practicing primary care NPs who care for women throughout their lives. NPs create strong patient relationships, provide safe clinical environments, and work with their patients on essential health promotion and disease prevention activities. This article outlined the common components of the WWV across all age groups, such as a comprehensive patient history, head to toe PE, health screening, health counseling and anticipatory guidance, as well as the key components that are unique to each age group. For additional resources for the WWV, see Table 7. Although guidelines and recommendations have been provided for the well-woman examination through these life stages, it is important to keep in mind the value and importance of individualizing care and considering each woman's unique needs, patient history, risks, social determinants of health, and PE findings when performing the annual WWV for women of all ages.

Disclosure

None of the authors have any affiliations with or involvement in any organization or entity with any financial interest (such as honoraria; educational grants; participation in speakers' bureaus; membership, employment, consultancies, stock ownership, or other equity interest; and expert testimony or patent-licensing arrangements), or nonfinancial interest (such as personal or professional relationships, affiliations, knowledge, or beliefs) in the subject matter or materials discussed in this article.

References

[1] Well-woman visit. American College of Obstetricians and Gynecologists (ACOG.org. 2018. Available at: https://www.acog.org/clinical/clinical-guidance/committee-opinion/articles/2018/10/well-woman-visit. Accessed September 15, 2021.

[2] Bickley LS. Bates' guide to physical examination and history taking. 12th edition. Philadelphia: Wolters Kluwer; 2017.

[3] Carr DD. Motivational interviewing supports patient-centered care and communication. J N Y State Nurses Assoc 2016;45(139):39–43. Available at: https://www.nysna.org/sites/default/files/attach/1142/2017/08/2017-08-01nysnaJournalv45n1.pdf#page=41. Accessed: September 15, 2021.

[4] McDonald EG, Dounaevskaia V, Lee TC. Inpatient attire: an opportunity to improve the patient experience. JAMA Intern Med 2014;174(11):1865–7.

[5] Effective patient–physician communication. Committee Opinion No. 587. ACOG.org. February 2014. Available at: https://www.acog.org/clinical/clinical-guidance/committee-opinion/articles/2014/02/effective-patient-physician-communication.   Accessed: September 15, 2021.

[6] Hashim MJ. Patient-centered communication: Basic skills. Am Fam Physician 2017;95(1): 29–34. Available at: https://www-aafp-org.proxy.lib.umich.edu/afp/2017/0101/p29.html. Accessed September 15, 2021.

[7] Collecting sexual orientation and gender identity information: importance of the collection and use of these data. Centers for Disease Control and Prevention; 2020. Available at: https://www.cdc.gov/hiv/clinicians/transforming-health/health-care-providers/collecting-sexual-orientation.html. Accessed September 15, 2021.

[8] Kuzma EK, Pardee M, Darling-Fisher CS. LGBT health: Creating safe spaces and caring for patients with cultural humility. J Am Assoc Nurs Pract 2019;31(3):167–74.

[9] Grasso C, Goldhammer H, Brown RJ, et al. Using sexual orientation and gender identity data in electronic health records to assess for disparities in preventive health screening services. Int J Med Inform 2020;142:104245.

[10] Sexual health questions to ask all patients. National Coalition for Sexual Health; 2021. Available at: https://nationalcoalitionforsexualhealth.org/tools/for-healthcare-providers/sexual-health-questions-to-ask-all-patients. Accessed September 15, 2021.

[11] McShane M, Perucho J, Olsakowski M, et al. Menstrual history-taking at annual well visits for adolescent girls. J Pediatr Adolesc Gynecol 2018;31(6):566–70.

[12] CODIERS SMASH FM (Flip cards). Chegg. 2021. Available at: https://www.chegg.com/flashcards/codiers-smash-fm-flip-cards-c704eed9-f519-48d6-b51d-fe8b32169c5d/deck. Accessed September 15, 2021.

[13] Questions you always ask to patients. The Student Doctor Network; 2013. Available at: https://forums.studentdoctor.net/threads/questions-you-always-ask-to-patients.975970/. Accessed September 15, 2021.

[14] Basile KC, Hertz MF, Back SE. Intimate partner violence and sexual violence victimization assessment instruments for use in healthcare settings: version 1. Atlanta (GA): Centers for Disease Control and Prevention, National Center for Injury Prevention and Control; 2007. Available at: https://www.cdc.gov/violenceprevention/pdf/ipv/ipvandsvscreening.pdf. Accessed September 15, 2021.

[15] Twenty things physicians and patients should question. Choosing Wisely. American Academy of Family Physicians. 2021. Available at: https://www.choosingwisely.org/societies/american-academy-of-family-physicians/. Accessed September 15, 2021.

[16] Don't require a pelvic exam or other physical exam to prescribe oral contraceptive medications. Choosing Wisely. 2021. American Academy of Family Physicians. Available at: https://www.choosingwisely.org/societies/american-academy-of-family-physicians/. Accessed September 15, 2021.

[17] Gregory KD, Chelmow D, Nelson HD, et al. Screening for anxiety in adolescent and adult women: A recommendation from the women's preventive services initiative. Annals of

Internal Medicine. Accessed September 15, 2021. Available at: https://doi.org/10.7326/M20-0580.

[18] Depression in adults: Screening. US Preventive Services Task Force. 2016. Available at: https://www.uspreventiveservicestaskforce.org/uspstf/document/RecommendationStatementFinal/depression-in-adults-screening. Accessed September 15, 2021.

[19] Depression in adolescents: AAP updates guidelines on diagnosis and treatment. Am Fam Physician 2018;98(7):462–3. Available at: https://www.aafp.org/afp/2018/1001/p462.html. Accessed September 15, 2021.

[20] Three tools for screening for social determinants of health. FPM. 2018. Available at: https://www.aafp.org/journals/fpm/blogs/inpractice/entry/social_determinants.html. Accessed September 15, 2021.

[21] Kuzma EK, Pardee M, Morgan A. Implementing patient-centered trauma-informed care for the perinatal nurse. J Perinat Neonatal Nurs 2020;34(4):E23–31.

[22] Lee EC. Adolescent preferences for topics addressed during well visits. WMJ 2017;116(4):210–4. Available at: https://wmjonline.org/wp-content/uploads/2017/116/4/210.pdf.

[23] Kuzma EK, Peters RM. Adolescent vulnerability, sexual health, and the NP's role in health advocacy. J Am Assoc Nurse Pract 2016;28(7):353–61.

[24] U.S. Supreme Court. Carey v. Population Services International. 9 Jun 1977. U S Rep U S Supreme Court. 1977;431:678-719.

[25] Sidorowicz K, Hair EC, Milot A. Assessing Bullying: A Guide for Out-of-School Time Program Practitioners. Child Trends. 2009. Available at: https://www.childtrends.org/wp-content/uploads/2009/10/child_trends-2009_10_29_rb_assessingbullying.pdf. Accessed September 15, 2021.

[26] David CG, Susan JC, Douglas KO. Screening for Adolescent Idiopathic Scoliosis: US Preventive Services Task Force Recommendation Statement. JAMA : The Journal of the American Medical Association, 2017. vol. 319, no. 2, United States: American Medical Association, pp. 165–72, doi:10.1001/jama.2017.19342.

[27] Screening recommendations and considerations referenced in treatment guidelines and original sources. Centers for Disease Control and Prevention. 2021. Available at: https://www.cdc.gov/std/treatment-guidelines/screening-recommendations.htm. Accessed September 15, 2021.

[28] Bright futures guidelines for health supervision of infants, children, and adolescents. Adolescent visits: 11 through 21 years. American Academy of Pediatrics. Available at: https://brightfutures.aap.org/Bright%20Futures%20Documents/BF4_AdolescenceVisits.pdf. Accessed September 19, 2021.

[29] Kudesia R, Talib HJ, Pollack SE. Fertility awareness counseling for adolescent girls; guiding conception: The right time, right weight, and right way. J Pediatr Adolesc Gynecol 2017;30(1):9–17.

[30] Curry S, Krist A, Owens D, et al. Behavioral weight loss interventions to prevent obesity-related morbidity and mortality in adults. JAMA 2018;320(11):1163.

[31] US Preventive Services Task Force, Krist AH, Davidson KW, et al. Screening for hypertension in adults: US Preventive Services Task Force Reaffirmation Recommendation Statement. JAMA 2021;325(16):1650–6.

[32] How and when to have your cholesterol checked. Centers for Disease Control and Prevention; 2021. Available at: https://www.cdc.gov/cholesterol/checked.htm. Accessed September 26, 2021.

[33] How to get your cholesterol tested. 2021. Available at: www.heart.org; https://www.heart.org/en/health-topics/cholesterol/how-to-get-your-cholesterol-tested. Accessed September 26, 2021.

[34] Patnode CD, Henderson JT, Coppola EL, et al. Interventions for tobacco cessation in adults, including pregnant persons: Updated evidence report and systematic review for the US Preventive Services Task Force. JAMA 2021;325(3):280–98.

[35] Jin J. Screening for cardiovascular disease risk with ECG. JAMA 2018;319(22):2346.

[36] Dyslipidemia management for cardiovascular disease prevention: Guidelines from the VA/ DoD. Am Fam Physician 2021;103(8):507–9. Available at: https://www.aafp.org/afp/ 2021/0415/p507.html.

[37] Marcus JZ, Cason P, Downs LS Jr, et al. The ASCCP Cervical Cancer Screening Task Force endorsement and opinion on the American Cancer Society updated cervical cancer screening guidelines. J Low Genit Tract Dis 2021;25(3):187–91.

[38] Fontham ETH, Wolf AMD, Church TR, et al. Cervical cancer screening for individuals at average risk: 2020 guideline update from the American Cancer Society. CA Cancer J Clin 2020;70(5):321–46.

[39] Shaukat A, Kahi CJ, Burke CA, et al. ACG Clinical Guidelines: Colorectal Cancer Screening 2021. Am J Gastroenterol 2021;116(3):458–79.

[40] US Preventive Services Task Force, Davidson KW, Barry MJ, et al. Screening for prediabetes and type 2 diabetes: US Preventive Services Task Force Recommendation Statement. JAMA 2021;326(8):736–43.

[41] US Preventive Services Task Force, Davidson KW, Barry MJ, et al. Screening for Gestational Diabetes: US Preventive Services Task Force Recommendation Statement. JAMA 2021;326(6):531–8.

[42] 2021 Coding guide screening for gestational diabetes mellitus. Women's Preventive Services Initiative (WPSI). Available at: https://www.womenspreventivehealth.org/wp-content/uploads/WPSI_ClinicalSummaryTables_DIGITAL.pdf. Accessed September 26, 2021.

[43] American Diabetes Association. 2. Classification and Diagnosis of Diabetes: Standards of Medical Care in Diabetes-2021 [published correction appears in Diabetes Care. 2021 Sep;44(9):2182]. Diabetes Care 2021;44(Suppl 1):S15–33.

[44] Ito Fukunaga M, Wiener RS, Slatore CG. The 2021 US Preventive Services Task Force recommendation on lung cancer screening: The more things stay the same…. JAMA Oncol 2021;7(5):684–6.

[45] Osteoporosis Prevention. Screening, and Diagnosis: ACOG Clinical Practice Guideline No. 1. Obstet Gynecol 2021;138(3):494–506.

[46] US Preventive Services Task Force. Screening for osteoporosis to prevent fractures. JAMA 2018;319(24):2521–31.

[47] FRAX: Fracture Risk Assessment Tool. Sheffield.ac.uk. 2008. Available at: https:// www.sheffield.ac.uk/FRAX/. Accessed September 25, 2021.

[48] US Preventive Services Task Force, Owens DK, Davidson KW, et al. Preexposure prophylaxis for the prevention of HIV Infection: US Preventive Services Task Force Recommendation Statement. JAMA 2019;321(22):2203–13.

[49] Johnson MM, Leachman SA, Aspinwall LG, et al. Skin cancer screening: Recommendations for data-driven screening guidelines and a review of the US Preventive Services Task Force controversy. Melanoma Manag 2017;4(1):13–37.

[50] Skin cancer: Screening. Final recommendation statement. US Preventive Services Task Force. 2016. Available at: https://www.uspreventiveservicestaskforce.org/uspstf/document/RecommendationStatementFinal/skin-cancer-screening. Accessed September 15, 2021.

[51] PDQ® Screening and Prevention Editorial Board. PDQ Skin Cancer Screening. Bethesda, MD: National Cancer Institute. Updated April 12, 2021. Available at: https://www.cancer.gov/types/skin/patient/skin-screening-pdq. Accessed September 15, 2021.

[52] Phipps MG, Son S, Zahn C, et al. Women's Preventive Services Initiative's Well-Woman Chart: A summary of preventive health recommendations for women. Obstet Gynecol 2019;134(3):465–9.

[53] O'Reilly N, Nelson HD, Conry JM, et al. Screening for urinary incontinence: A recommendation from the Women's Preventive Services Initiative. Ann Intern Med 2018;169(5): 320–8.

[54] Mehta S, Wallace S, Desrosiers L, et al. Using the questionnaire for urinary incontinence diagnosis as screening tool in low resource settings. Am J Obstet Gynecol 2017;216(3): S610–611doi.

[55] Committee on Gynecologic Practice American Society for Reproductive Medicine, Breitkopf DM, Hill M. Pre-pregnancy counseling. Committee opinion number 762. Published January 2019 (Reaffirmed 2020). Available at: https://www.acog.org/clinical/clinical-guidance/committee-opinion/articles/2019/01/prepregnancy-counseling.

[56] Seematter-Bagnoud L, Büla C. Brief assessments and screening for geriatric conditions in older primary care patients: A pragmatic approach. Public Health Rev 2018;39:8.

[57] Heflin MT. Geriatric health maintenance. In: Schmader KE, Givens J, section, editors. UpToDate Inc; 2021. Available at: https://www.uptodate.com/contents/geriatric-health-maintenance. Accessed September 2, 2021.

[58] Elmore JG, Lee CI. Screening for breast cancer: Strategies and recommendations. In: Aronson MD, Kunins L, section, editors. UpToDate Inc.; 2021. Available at: https://www.uptodate.com/contents/screening-for-breast-cancer-strategies-and-recommendations?topicRef=3017&source=see_link. Accessed September 20, 2021.

[59] Colorectal cancer: Screening. Final recommendation statement. US Preventive Services Task Force. 2021. Available at: https://www.uspreventiveservicestaskforce.org/uspstf/recommendation/colorectal-cancer-screening. Accessed September 15, 2021.

[60] Medicare wellness visits. Medicare Learning Network. Available at: https://www.cms.gov/Outreach-and-Education/Medicare-Learning-Network-MLN/MLNProducts/preventive-services/medicare-wellness-visits.html. Accessed September 15, 2021.

[61] Ward KT, Rubin DB. Comprehensive geriatric assessment. In: Schmader KE, Givens J, section, editors. UpToDate Inc.; 2021. Available at: https://www.uptodate.com/contents/comprehensive-geriatric-assessment?topicRef=3017&source=see_link#H5. Accessed September 15, 2021.

[62] Kiel DP. Falls in older persons: Risk factors and patient evaluation. In: Schmader KE, Givens J, section, editors. UpToDate Inc.; 2021. Available at: https://www.uptodate.com/contents/falls-in-older-persons-risk-factors-and-patient-evaluation?sectionName=FALLS%20RISK%20ASSESSMENT&topicRef=3009&anchor=H21&source=see_link#H21. Accessed September 15, 2021.

[63] Caregiving US. Department of Health and Human Services. National Institute on Aging. Available at: https://www.nia.nih.gov/health/caregiving/advance-care-planning. Accessed September 15, 2021.

Recurrent Vulvovaginal Candidiasis: Implications for Practice

Check for updates

Mary Lauren Pfieffer, DNP, FNP-BC

Vanderbilt University School of Nursing, 461 21st Avenue South, FH 354, Nashville, TN 37240, USA

Keywords

- Vulvovaginal candidiasis (VVC) • Recurrent vulvovaginal candidiasis
- Chronic vulvovaginal candidiasis • Recurrent vaginal conditions
- Candida albicans

Key points

- Vulvovaginal candidiasis is caused by overgrowth of *Candida* yeast. Differentiating vulvovaginal candidiasis, recurrent vulvovaginal candidiasis, and chronic vulvovaginal candidiasis is imperative for treatment and improved quality of life for patient.
- Clinical presentation depends on the chronicity of the condition but could include itching, irritation, discharge, odor, soreness, dyspareunia, cyclicity of symptoms, and vaginal swelling.
- Diagnostic tests include vaginal pH, bedside testing with 10% potassium hydroxide and saline, vaginal culture, nucleic acid amplification tests, and also DNA polymerase chain reaction tests.
- Treatment of vulvovaginal candidiasis depends on the chronicity but can be oral or topical with varying duration.

CASE

L.P. is a 32-year-old woman who presents to clinic with vaginal symptoms that have occurred for the past week with worsening symptoms over the past 3 days: vaginal itching, dyspareunia, and vaginal discharge. This is the fourth time she has had these complaints this past year. She self-treated once with over-the-counter cream but came in for evaluation and treatment 2 times. She has a history of polycystic ovarian syndrome (PCOS) and has had some urinary leakage since her last child. Patient states that the continuation and recurrence of symptoms over the past year has been hard on her sexual

E-mail address: mary.pfieffer@vanderbilt.edu

https://doi.org/10.1016/j.yfpn.2021.12.006
2589-420X/22/© 2021 Elsevier Inc. All rights reserved.

relationship and she lacks self-confidence. She has had to miss some work related to the severity of symptoms. She reports that symptoms recur when she resumes physical exercise. The recurrent symptoms have also affected her enough that she has begun missing work. All of these issues have led to depression symptoms. She has a 5-year-old and a 9-month-old at home. She reports being in a monogamous relationship. She takes Zovia 1/35 birth control (ethinyl estradiol and ethynodiol diacetate), Zoloft (Sertraline), 50 mg, PO QD, and a prenatal vitamin. She was on Augmentin (amoxicillin and clavulanate potassium) 2 months ago for a sinus infection. Otherwise, no other medications. Patient states she has no known drug allergies. Family history is significant for diabetes mellitus type 2 in her father and both of her paternal grandparents. Her maternal grandmother had hypertension, hypothyroidism, and breast cancer. No other significant family history.

L.P.'s vitals indicate that her blood pressure, pulse, and temperature are all within normal limits. Her body mass index (BMI) is 35. Physical examination is revealing for erythematous vulva and vulvar excoriation present. Speculum examination shows scant white discharge in vaginal vault. No vaginal atrophy is present. Differential diagnoses considered are bacterial vaginosis, vulvovaginal candidiasis (VVC), recurrent VVC, lichen sclerosis, and atrophic vaginitis. Vaginal pH is normal. Microscopy with potassium hydroxide (KOH) is revealing for budding yeast but no clue cells. Vaginal culture is obtained and sent for processing.

Differentials were ruled out visualizing the budding yeast with no clue cells on microscopy; this rules out bacterial vaginosis, as there are no clue cells. Lichen sclerosis is ruled out by the speculum examination revealing white discharge, and there are no fissures or thin, parchment-like skin present. Atrophic vaginitis is ruled out, as she has white discharge versus yellow. Her age does not make her susceptible to atrophic vaginitis and she does not have a history of surgery that would remove her ovaries. She is not on any medications to make her more susceptible to this condition, such as one of the new birth control gels that have a side effect of vaginal burning and itching. Vaginal atrophy is not present, which also rules out atrophic vaginitis.

The diagnosis is recurrent VVC based on assessment, vaginal pH, budding yeast seen with microscopy, and frequency of symptoms over the past year. She is prescribed induction therapy of fluconazole, 150 mg, every 72 hours for a total of 3 doses to be followed with maintenance therapy using fluconazole, 150 mg, once a week for 6 months. Three days later culture results revealed for Candida albicans, which reinforces treatment prescribed. Patient education was given to change clothes after exercise and discontinue using scented soap surrounding vaginal area.

VVC is a frequent vaginal infection affecting women worldwide. VVC is an acute inflammatory condition of the vulva and vaginal mucosa correlated to overgrowth of *Candida* yeast [1]. Seventy-five percent of women will experience VVC during their lifetime [2]. Forty percent of women presenting to a primary care office with vaginal complaints are diagnosed with VVC [3,4]. Total outpatient cost burden of VVC in the United States is roughly $368 million a year [5]. The economic burden related to productivity loss with VVC is roughly $1 billion [2].

Recurrent VVC is reoccurring VVC roughly 4 times a year despite treatment. Although patients with VVC have asymptomatic periods between treatments, the duration will vary with patients when they do have symptoms; for example, some will have episodes from 1 to 2 years or 4 to 5 years [6]. The incidence of recurrent VVC is roughly 138 million women a year and affects 372 million women during a lifetime [7]. Recurrent VVC has the highest prevalence in the 25- to 34-year age group [7]. The economic burden of recurrent VVC is high with a potential lost productivity at 1 to $14 billion a year [2,7].

Chronic VVC is a newer term seen in the literature. In chronic VVC, patients have chronic symptoms of VVC, and the only time patients are asymptomatic is while on treatment [8]; this varies from recurrent VVC where there are periods of being asymptomatic between treatment [8]. Prevalence and epidemiology studies need to be completed for chronic VVC to show the impact this condition has on patients worldwide.

PATHOPHYSIOLOGY

Ninety percent of the time VVC and recurrent VVC is caused by the fungal pathogen *Candida albicans*, but it can similarly be caused by other *nonalbicans Candida*, such as *Candida glabrata*, *Candida krusei*, *Candida famata*, and *Candida tropicalis* [7,9]. *Candida* migrates from the lower gastrointestinal tract to the vagina and is present in a large percentage of healthy, asymptomatic women [6,10]. *Candida* then colonizes in the vagina and binds to the epithelial cells [6]. This colonization can be enhanced by estrogen, therefore increasing after menarche and declining after menopause [6]. The vaginal ecosystem is composed of many microorganisms to combat *Candida* overgrowth including *Lactobacilli* and other antibacterial compounds [3,11].

Several factors can generate *Candida* overgrowth and trigger an inflammatory response in the vagina causing VVC and recurrent VVC [6] (Table 1). The initial risk is related to estrogen: *Candida* is increased when there is more

Table 1
Risk factors vulvovaginal candidiasis

Comorbidities	Contributing Factors	Medications
Uncontrolled diabetes mellitus	Sexual activity	Topical steroid use
Obesity	Immunosuppression	Hormone replacement therapy
Vulvar disease	Pregnancy	Recent antibiotic use
Lichen sclerosis	High carbohydrate dietary intake	Contraceptive devices
—	Douching	Intrauterine devices (IUDs)
—	Feminine hygiene products	—

Data from Refs [6,10,11,13]

estrogen [11]. Therefore, when patients are taking oral contraceptives, hormone replacement therapy, or are pregnant the risk is increased [11]. The second most common risk for *Candida* relates to glycogen. *Candida* receives nutrition from glycogen. Consequently, patients who are obese, consuming high carbohydrate diet, diabetic, or are using topical or oral steroids are at risk for *Candida* overgrowth [11]. Antibiotic use decreases vaginal lactobacilli, causing *Candida* overgrowth [10,11]. Regardless if antibiotics are oral or topical, *Candida* overgrowth can still be triggered [10]. Although these risk factors can lead to *Candida* infections, there is not always a causal relationship.

Studies are needed to identify specific pathophysiological contributors to recurrent VVC and chronic VVC, as there is relatively little information available on this in the literature. The terms candidiasis and candidosis will both be seen in the literature, as inflammation is not always present with VVC and recurrent VVC [11]. A debatable element with VVC and recurrent VVC is that sometimes it is categorized with sexually transmitted infections, as it can be obtained from sexual activities [11]. For example, semen causes changes in the vaginal pH that can predispose to *Candida* overgrowth in the vagina [11].

A recent study indicated the absence of vaginal biofilms with *Candida* infections [12]. Vaginal biofilms are clusters of microorganisms that attach to the vaginal epithelium. Patients who have biofilms are generally more difficult to treat, as organisms are harder to penetrate. Patients with bacterial vaginosis were shown to have vaginal biofilms [12]. This new information helps to distinguish between bacterial vaginosis (BV) and Candida infections and aids in the misdiagnosing of VVC, recurrent VVC, and chronic VVC [12]. Future research may offer methods to improve distinguishing BV from *Candida* infections and to help establish protective vaginal biofilms.

CLINICAL PRESENTATION

Patients with VVC often present with the hallmark signs of *Candida* overgrowth: vaginal itching, vaginal irritation, and white discharge [6] (Table 2). Patients often report itching on the vulva [6]. The itching can range in severity from mild to incapacitating [3]. Vaginal irritation can cause dysuria, dyspareunia, and overall vaginal discomfort [13]. Vaginal discharge with VVC has been discussed most frequently as thick and white but can also range from watery to thick in consistency [2]. The vaginal discharge is a nonspecific finding [6]. Odor is not always present in these patients but is usually nonoffensive if present, unlike BV, which often has an amine odor [2]. Some patients reveal that symptoms increase or become worse the week before menses [2].

There are 3 types of VVC: VVC, recurrent, and chronic. A single episode or infrequent episodes of VVC are diagnosed and treated with no follow-up or maintenance therapy required. What differentiates VVC from recurrent VVC is that recurrence of symptoms occurs 3 times or more over a 12-month period [6]. Patients with chronic VVC present with many of the same symptoms but with increased chronicity. Chronic VVC is a condition of chronic, nonspecific, and nonerosive vulvovaginitis that includes several of the

Table 2
Clinical signs and symptoms of vulvovaginal candidiasis

External Symptoms	Vaginal Symptoms
Burning	Dyspareunia
Excoriation	Discharge: thick white to watery in consistency
Fissures	Dryness
Itching	Dysuria
Edema	Erythema
—	Odor

Data from Denning DW, Kneale M, Sobel JD, Rautemaa-Richardson R. Global burden of recurrent vulvovaginal candidiasis: a systematic review. The Lancet Infectious Diseases. 2018;18(11):e339-e347. DOI: 10.1016/S1473-3099(18)30103-8; and Donders GGG, Grinceviciene S, Bellen G, Ruban K. Is multiple-site colonization with Candida spp. related to inadequate response to individualized fluconazole maintenance therapy in women with recurrent Candida vulvovaginitis? Diagnostic Microbiology and Infectious Disease. 2018;92(3):226-229. https://doi.org/10.1016/j.diagmicrobio.2018.05.024.

following characteristics: vaginal soreness, dyspareunia, present or history of positive vaginal swab, previous antifungal medication for VVC, exacerbation of symptoms with antibiotic use, cyclicity of VVC symptoms, vaginal swelling, and vaginal discharge [6,8]. Patients with recurrent VVC and chronic VVC may have *Candida* in extragenital sites; therefore, assessment of urine, perineum, and the anus is encouraged [14].

Patients with recurrent VVC and chronic VVC struggle with psychosocial and psychological problems due to the chronicity of the condition. Anxiety and depression are often seen with patients [15]. These patients also tend to lack self-confidence and self-esteem related to the continued need for treatment despite lifestyle changes [7]. Patients with recurrent VVC and chronic VVC are not able to carry out physical activities as often related to vaginal discomfort [7,9]. And lastly these patients struggle with intimate relationships, as there is misconception that this is a sexually transmitted disease [7,9,11].

Several of the presenting clinical symptoms of VVC and recurrent VVC overlap with other vaginal conditions, so paying close attention to history and performing an examination are important for diagnosis [6]. Many patients self-treat with over-the-counter meds, and sometimes they have self-treated multiple times before coming in for evaluation, which is why taking a detailed history on what they have tried at home is important in the patient history as well. It is important that diagnosis should not be based on examination findings alone. Patients often come in self-diagnosed with VVC and that can sway providers' diagnosis [6]. VVC is commonly underdiagnosed or misdiagnosed [6,9].

DIAGNOSIS

On examination, patients with VVC and recurrent VVC will often have erythematous vulva and labia [2]. There also may be fissures and excoriation present [16]. Cervical examination of a patient with VVC and recurrent VVC is normal but thick, white discharge may be present in the vaginal vault [2]. Because clinical findings can vary, diagnosis should not be based on examination findings alone [6].

There are other differentials to consider with evaluating a patient for VVC, recurrent VVC, and chronic VVC. Some differentials to consider are lichen simplex chronicus, lichen sclerosis, vulvodynia, and vulvar contact dermatitis. There are key physical examination findings to help differentiate. Lichen simplex chronicus presents with dry plaques and thickened lesions with erythema related to pruritis [17]. These plaques can be in many areas on the body but are frequently seen on head, neck, arms, scalp, and genitals, as these places are easier to reach [17]. Lichen simplex chronicus is not associated with vaginal discharge [17]. Lichen sclerosis is another common differential to consider. Vulvar lichen sclerosis is the term identifying the condition more specific to the vagina [18]. Clinical presentation of this would potentially include waxy, white plaques, bruising, and changes in pigmentation [18]. It can affect many areas of the vaginal but rarely involves vaginal mucosa and also is not associated with vaginal discharge [18]. VVC, recurrent VVC, and chronic VVC can cause vulvar pain related to pruritis; therefore, the differential of vulvodynia needs to be considered. Vulvodynia on examination could reveal fissures and vulvar inflammation, but discharge is not seen with this clinical condition [19]. Lastly, vulvar contact dermatitis needs to be considered in these patients. Patients with vulvar contact dermatitis have erythematous, demarcated plaques in area that was in contact with external agent [20]. This plaque can be vesicular or scaly in nature [20]. There is no discharge associated with vulvar contact dermatitis [20]. Ruling out these differentials is important to patients with VVC, recurrent VVC, and chronic VVC, so they are not misdiagnosed and underdiagnosed with the appropriate condition.

Diagnosis of VVC and recurrent VVC can be confirmed with several diagnostic tests. First consider the pH. The pH in a patient with VVC is normal, whereas it is elevated in patients with bacterial vaginosis or other vaginitis diagnoses [11]. Diagnosis cannot be made on pH alone, as there can be mixed infections present in vagina [2,11]. Bedside laboratory tests can be performed to confirm VVC: 10% KOH and saline. Patients with VVC will have hyphae, pseudohyphae, or budding yeast under microscopy [16]. Patients with VVC will not have clue cells that would distinguish a patient with bacterial vaginosis [2]. Health care providers are not always trained with microscopy skills, and furthermore it is often replaced with other diagnostic tests [6].

If pH and microscopy are normal but patient examination is suspicious of VVC, then culture needs to be obtained [6]. Vaginal culture has been the gold standard of diagnosis VVC for some time [6]. Culture should always be obtained in patients with recurrent VVC and chronic VVC to identify non-*Candida* albicans causes of their condition [16]. If culture returns with *Candida* but patient is asymptomatic, treatment should not be prescribed, as roughly 10% of women have *Candida* in normal vaginal flora [21]. The disadvantages of vaginal culture are the time it takes for results and the lack of *Candida* identification with certain cultures [22].

There are newer diagnostic tests, and it is unclear the trajectory these tests will have in diagnosing VVC, recurrent VVC, and chronic VVC. There are a few nucleic acid amplification tests (NAATs) that can be used to detect *Candida* [22]. The DNA polymerase chain reaction (PCR) test is reliable in detecting microorganisms of *Candida* [23]. Results of the PCR can be received in several days [6]. Treatment does not need to be prescribed until results are received. Treating before results can lead to unnecessary and improper treatment. If patient is uncomfortable, giving supportive treatments will help until test results. Reassurance that laboratory results are typically back in 24 to 48 hours can give patients some comfort. If patient is seen before a weekend and health care provider highly suspects VVC, then there is an option to treat the symptoms and wait on the result but waiting on result is best practice.

NAAT and PCR tests are more expensive than the traditional culture [23]. Some examples of these NAATs are BD Affirm, Gen-Probe, Aptima, and the BD MAX Vaginal Panel test. NAATs are the standard of care in many places versus culture for several reasons: lack of microscopy equipment in office, lack of providers trained in microscopy if available, lack of sensitivity with culture, lack of *Candida* identification with culture, and improved objective diagnosis of vaginal infection with NAATs [22].

TREATMENT

Topical agents are useful in treating VVC (Table 3). Over-the-counter versions of azole intravaginal creams are mainly what is used for treatment [16,24]. Treatment duration depends on cream formulation, strength, and severity of patient symptoms [16]. If the patient has VVC, generally a 7-day course is sufficient [16]. If the patient has recurrent VVC or chronic VVC, a 14-day course of topical azole can be helpful [24].

Oral agents are effective in treating VVC as well. Generally, a single dose of fluconazole, 150 mg, is used for treatment of VVC [24]. If VVC symptoms are severe, increasing treatment duration to fluconazole, 150 mg, given every 72 hours for a total of 3 doses should suffice [24].

Recurrent VVC and chronic VVC treatment can alter in duration and depends on the type of *Candida* infection (Table 4). It is important that a culture is obtained to ensure eradication of specific *Candida* overgrowth [24]. Topical azoles, boric acid, topical amphotericin B, or oral voriconazole can be useful for recurrent VVC and chronic VVC [6,25]. An induction and maintenance phase of these medications is used for treatment [6]. Up to 50% of patients will have recurrence of symptoms after cessation of maintenance phase of treatment [6,22]. If reoccurrence occurs after initial induction and maintenance, then reinduction is recommended with alternative medication followed by 6 to 12 months of weekly fluconazole, 150 mg [6]. The average length of maintenance therapy is 9 months [26].

Table 3
Topical treatment for vulvovaginal candidiasis

Over-the-Counter	Dosage	Pregnancy and Breastfeeding
Clotrimazole 1%/2% Cream	1%: use daily for 7–14 d 2%: use daily for 3 d	Safe to use: recommended 7-d treatment
Miconazole 2%/4% Cream 100 mg/200 mg Suppository	2%: use daily for 7 d 4%: use daily for 3 d Suppositories: 3–7 d	Safe to use: recommended 7-d treatment
Tioconazole 6.5% Cream	Intravaginally in single application	Safe to use
Prescription		
Butoconazole 2% Cream	Intravaginally in single application	Safe to use
Terconazole 0.4%/0.8% Cream 80 mg Suppository	0.4%: use daily for 7 d 0.8%: use daily for 3 d Suppository: one daily for 3 d	Safe to use: recommended 7-d treatment

Topical "azoles" are safe to use and recommended for first-line treatment of pregnancy and breastfeeding.
Data from Charifa A, Badri T, Harris BW. Lichen Simplex Chronicus. [Updated 2020 Aug 10]. In: Stat-Pearls [Internet]. Treasure Island (FL): StatPearls Publishing; 2020 Jan.

There are nonpharmacologic treatment options for treatment of VVC, recurrent VVC, and chronic VVC. Probiotics with Lactobacillus have been used as alternative method for treatment, although research is not as established [6,27]. Lactobacillus is thought to reduce *Candida* virulence and improve vaginal epithelial defense [6]. Boric acid vaginal suppositories have been shown to be effective for treatment of VVC/recurrent VVC/chronic VVC [6,16,24]. Generally, a 600 mg boric acid vaginal suppository is prescribed once a day for 14 days. If symptoms come back after cessation of treatment, a culture is needed to determine *Candida* species; however, maintenance boric acid suppositories can be used [6,16,24]. Not every pharmacy will carry boric acid; therefore, this may require a prescription be sent to a compounding pharmacy to be filled. Patients living in rural areas may have more difficulty accessing boric acid or a compounding pharmacy.

SPECIAL POPULATIONS
Pregnancy and breastfeeding
There are some patients who need special consideration when treating VVC. Patients who are pregnant are treated with topical azole treatment, and these topical agents are used for 7 days [16,28]. Oral treatment with fluconazole is contraindicated in pregnancy [16]. Azoles are secreted in milk; therefore, patients who are breastfeeding need alternative treatment.

Human immunodeficiency virus and diabetes
Patients with human immunodeficiency virus (HIV) have a greater tendency to colonization of *Candida* [16]. Treating HIV-infected patient with VVC is the

Table 4
Treatment of recurrent vulvovaginal candidiasis and chronic vulvovaginal candidiasis

Candida Species Type	Medication	Therapy Duration	Pregnancy and Breastfeeding
Candida albicans, Candida tropicalis, Candida parapsilosis	Fluconazole, 150 mg	Induction: 150 mg q 72 h for 3 doses Maintenance: 150 mg q weekly for 6 mo	Pregnancy: avoid in first trimester. Lowest duration possible. Breastfeeding: safe to use
	Itraconazole, 200 mg	Induction: 200 mg bid × 3 d Maintenance: 200 mg/d for 6 mo	Pregnancy: avoid in first trimester Breastfeeding: not recommended
	Clotrimazole 1%/2% Miconazole 2%/4% Tioconazole 6.5%/0.4% Terconazole 0.8% vaginal cream/89 mg vaginal suppository Butoconazole 2%	Induction: cream duration depends on strength and severity of symptoms Maintenance: One suppository once weekly for 6 mo	See Table 3
Candida glabrata	Boric acid vaginal suppository/capsule 600 mg	Induction: one suppository daily for 14 d Maintenance: no data to support	Contraindicated in pregnancy and breastfeeding
	Nystatin–100,000-U vaginal suppository	Induction: one suppository per vagina for 14 d Maintenance: should be considered	Safe to use in pregnancy and breastfeeding
Azole-resistant Candida species	Boric acid vaginal suppository/capsule 600 mg	Induction: one suppository daily for 14 d Maintenance: no data to support	Contraindicated in pregnancy and breastfeeding

(continued on next page)

Table 4
(continued)

Candida Species Type	Medication	Therapy Duration	Pregnancy and Breastfeeding
	Nystatin–100,000-U vaginal suppository	*Induction:* one suppository per vagina for 14 d *Maintenance:* should be considered	Safe to use in pregnancy and breastfeeding
	Amphotericin B vaginal cream/suppositories 5%–10%	Suppositories used nightly for 14 d	May use second line for pregnancy and breastfeeding
	Flucytosine cream 17%	One vaginal application, nightly for 14 d	Avoid in pregnancy and breastfeeding

Topical "azoles" are recommended first line in pregnancy and breastfeeding. May consider fluconazole, 150 mg, one time if symptoms do not resolve. Only use oral "azoles" after first trimester.
Data from Refs [6,16,24]

same as treating a noninfected patient [21,28]. It is essential to treat immuno-compromised patients with a longer duration of treatment, generally for 7 to 14 days [16]. Diabetes mellitus and HIV can lead to patients having VVC, recurrent VVC, and chronic VVC; therefore, if patients have other risk factors, screening for those conditions may be appropriate [25].

Transwomen care
Transwomen who have had vaginoplasty can have candidiasis, and it is termed neovaginal candidiasis [29]. Patients often present with neovaginal discharge, odor, and pruritis [29]. Treatment of neovaginal candidiasis has been effective with miconazole, either topically or in a vaginal capsule [29]. More research needs to be done in this patient population, as although it is not a frequent condition seen in transwomen, it can cause discomfort to which treatment is necessary [29].

Other special populations
In VVC, recurrent VVC, and chronic VVC health care providers would only need to consider treatment of sexual partners if male partner is symptomatic with balanitis, as this can be caused by *Candida* infection [16]. Oral contraceptives can increase estrogen, therefore triggering *Candida*, so cessation of these or switching to a nonestrogen formulation of birth control may help eradicate *Candida* [29]. Health care providers need to be mindful of treating patients with azoles if they also take anticoagulants and anticonvulsants [11].

PSYCHOSOCIAL AND MENTAL HEALTH
An important piece of treatment is for providers to remember the psychosocial and potential mental health concerns. Screening for anxiety and depression should be done with these patients, particularly with patients experiencing chronic and recurrent VVC, as these can be very challenging on patients [15]. An important part of taking a good history would be to include asking the patient about how the symptoms or diagnosis affects their life in terms of job, self-esteem, intimate relationships, and physical activity. Discussing these daily activities of living may help identify some potential areas of concern as well as or need for some type of referral [7,9].

PATIENT EDUCATION
Patient education is important with patients with VVC. Educating patients that this is not a sexually transmitted disease is important for sexual health [7,9,11]. Intravaginal azole creams can weaken latex condoms, as they are oil based; therefore, educating about backup birth control is important [15]. Backup birth control education is not needed if patients are on oral contraceptives, as there is not any interaction with medication.

Patients with VVC, recurrent VVC, and chronic VVC need to abstain from sexual activity until symptoms resolve for best treatment. Physical activity can continue but encourage patients to change out of tight exercise ware and shower after exercise. For patients who require treatment, they should be encouraged to follow-up in 72 hours if symptoms are not improved or if symptoms worsen with treatment. Patients with recurrent and chronic VVC require follow-up to ensure that *Candida* is eradicated.

Although lacking in rigor, there has been some literature related to lowering sugar and carbohydrate intake to improve VVC symptoms and treatment [6]. More research is needed on the effect glucose consumption has on VVC. If a patient has a concern with this aspect, consider offering a referral for a nutrition consultation, particularly if they have a history of PCOS or elevated BMI. If the patient loses weight, insulin resistance and PCOS symptoms may improve.

SUMMARY

L.P.'s case is very straightforward for VVC but due to the frequency of symptoms over the past year and Candida albicans seen in culture, she was diagnosed with recurrent VVC. Patient education is very important for these patients, especially due to the psychosocial impact the patient experiences. After maintenance therapy, L.P.'s recurrent VVC symptoms are not currently present.

Women's health care providers will encounter VVC and recurrent VVC diagnoses frequently in primary care. Confirming diagnosis with vaginal culture can guarantee Candida type and help with treatment, as misdiagnosis happens frequently. Another way of improving misdiagnosis and underdiagnosis of VVC and recurrent VVC is having more providers proficient with vaginal microscopy. Additional training would enhance this specialized skill. Ensuring that providers are aware of treatment of recurrent VVC is important for the psychological impact patients confront with this diagnosis.

References

[1] Fidel PL, Barousse M, Espinosa T, et al. An intravaginal live Candida challenge in humans leads to new hypotheses for the immunopathogenesis of vulvovaginal candidiasis. Infect Immun 2004;72(5):2939–46.
[2] Sobel JD. Vulvovaginal candidosis. Lancet 2007;369(9577):1961–71.
[3] Ilkit M, Guzel AB. The epidemiology, pathogenesis, and diagnosis of vulvovaginal candidosis: a mycological perspective. Crit Rev Microbiol 2011;37(3):250–61.
[4] Benedict K, Jackson BR, Chiller T, et al. Estimation of Direct Healthcare Costs of Fungal Diseases in the United States. Clin Infect Dis 2019;68(11):1791–7.
[5] Sobel JD. Recurrent vulvovaginal candidiasis. Am J Obstet Gynecol 2016;214(1):15–21.
[6] Denning DW, Kneale M, Sobel JD, et al. Global burden of recurrent vulvovaginal candidiasis: a systematic review. Lancet Infect Dis 2018;18(11):e339–47.
[7] Hong E, Dixit S, Fidel PL, et al. Vulvovaginal Candidiasis as a Chronic Disease: Diagnostic Criteria and Definition. J Lower Genital Tract Dis 2014;18(1):31–8.
[8] Blostein F, Levin-Sparenberg E, Wagner J, et al. Recurrent vulvovaginal candidiasis. Ann Epidemiol 2017;27(9):575–82.e573.
[9] Shukla A, Sobel JD. Vulvovaginitis Caused by Candida Species Following Antibiotic Exposure. Curr Infect Dis Rep 2019;21(11):44.
[10] Vieira-Baptista P, Bornstein J. Candidiasis, bacterial vaginosis. *Vulvar disease*, 167. Breaking the Myths; 2019; https://doi.org/10.1007/978-3-319-61621-6_24.
[11] Swidsinski A, Guschin A, Tang Q, et al. Vulvovaginal candidiasis: histologic lesions are primarily polymicrobial and invasive and do not contain biofilms. Am J Obstet Gynecol 2019;220(1):91.e1–8.

[12] Yano J, Sobel JD, Nyirjesy P, et al. Current patient perspectives of vulvovaginal candidiasis: incidence, symptoms, management and post-treatment outcomes. BMC Women's Health 2019;19(1):48.

[13] Donders GGG, Grinceviciene S, Bellen G, et al. Is multiple-site colonization with Candida spp. related to inadequate response to individualized fluconazole maintenance therapy in women with recurrent Candida vulvovaginitis? Diagn Microbiol Infect Dis 2018;92(3): 226–9.

[14] Aballéa S, Guelfucci F, Wagner J, et al. Subjective health status and health-related quality of life among women with Recurrent Vulvovaginal Candidosis (RVVC) in Europe and the USA. Health Qual Life Outcomes 2013;11(1):169.

[15] Itriyeva K. Evaluation of vulvovaginitis in the adolescent patient. Curr Probl Pediatr Adolesc Health Care 2020;50(7):100836.

[16] Charifa A, Badri T, Harris BW. Lichen Simplex Chronicus. In: StatPearls. Treasure Island (FL): StatPearls Publishing; 2020.

[17] Krapf JM, Mitchell L, Holton MA, et al. Vulvar Lichen Sclerosus: Current Perspectives. Int J Womens Health 2020;12:11–20.

[18] Stenson AL. Vulvodynia: Diagnosis and Management. Obstet Gynecol Clin North Am 2017;44(3):493–508.

[19] Pichardo-Geisinger R. Atopic and Contact Dermatitis of the Vulva. Obstet Gynecol Clin North Am 2017;44(3):371–8.

[20] Workowski KA, Bolan GA. Sexually transmitted diseases treatment guidelines, 2015. MMWR Recommendations Rep Morbidity mortality weekly Rep Recommendations Rep 2015;64(RR-03):1.

[21] Schwebke JR, Taylor SN, Ackerman R, et al. Clinical Validation of the Aptima Bacterial Vaginosis and Aptima Candida/Trichomonas Vaginitis Assays: Results from a Prospective Multicenter Clinical Study. J Clin Microbiol 2020;58(2):e01619–43.

[22] Sobel J, Akins RA. The Role of PCR in the Diagnosis of Candida Vulvovaginitis—a New Gold Standard? Curr Infect Dis Rep 2015;17(6):33.

[23] Pappas PG, Kauffman CA, Andes DR, et al. Clinical Practice Guideline for the Management of Candidiasis: 2016 Update by the Infectious Diseases Society of America. Clin Infect Dis 2016;62(4):e1–50.

[24] Zuckerman A, Romano M. Clinical Recommendation: Vulvovaginitis. J Pediatr Adolesc Gynecol 2016;29(6):673–9.

[25] Crouss T, Sobel JD, Smith K, et al. Long-Term Outcomes of Women With Recurrent Vulvovaginal Candidiasis After a Course of Maintenance Antifungal Therapy. J Low Genit Tract Dis 2018;22(4):382–6.

[26] Watson CJ, Pirotta M, Myers SP. Use of complementary and alternative medicine in recurrent vulvovaginal candidiasis–results of a practitioner survey. Complement Ther Med 2012;20(4):218–21.

[27] Centers for Disease Control and Prevention. Division of STD Prevention, National Center for HIV/AIDS, Viral Hepatitis, STD, and TB Prevention, Centers for Disease Control and Prevention. Vulvovaginal Candidiasis. 2015. Available at: https://www.cdc.gov/std/tg2015/candidiasis.htm. Accessed October 1, 2020.

[28] de Haseth KB, Buncamper ME, Özer M, et al. Symptomatic Neovaginal Candidiasis in Transgender Women After Penile Inversion Vaginoplasty: A Clinical Case Series of Five Consecutive Patients. Transgend Health 2018;3(1):105–8.

[29] Martin Lopez JE. Candidiasis (vulvovaginal). BMJ Clin Evid 2015;2015:0815.

Genitourinary Syndrome of Menopause

Assessment and Management Options

Laura C. Ford, PhD, RN, CNP

Western Michigan University, 8060 Talaria Terrace, Kalamazoo, MI 49009, USA

Keywords

- Genitourinary syndrome of menopause • GSM • Vulvovaginal atrophy
- Postmenopause atrophy • Sexual dysfunction of menopause

Key points

- Genitourinary syndrome of menopause (GSM) is a common disorder, experienced to some degree by more than 80% of menopausal women.
- Pharmacologic and lifestyle changes can help maintain function and reduce symptoms associated with this disorder.
- The primary care provider of a menopausal woman can assess the impact of endocrine loss on genital tissue and sexual function and begin to address the symptoms.
- Sexual function in women is multifactorial and addressing vaginal lubrication with the presence of pain or discomfort may help the menopausal patient maintain their relationship intimacy.

INTRODUCTION

Genitourinary syndrome of menopause (GSM) is a hypoestrogenic condition inclusive for complaints of genital discomfort, sexual dysfunction, and urinary signs and symptoms. This differs from vulvovaginal atrophy because it is inclusive of urinary complaints of incontinence, altered bladder capacity, and change in the urinary and vaginal microbiome [1]. The GSM condition was a term introduced in 2014 by the North American Menopause Society (NAMS) and the International Society for the Study of Women's Sexual Health [2–4]. This article educates the primary care clinician providing women's health care to enhance diagnosis and treatment of GSM because "it is essential to

E-mail address: Lauraford57@att.net

https://doi.org/10.1016/j.yfpn.2021.12.007

recognize and treat this syndrome in order to restore the vaginal and vulvar epithelium and ultimately improve quality of life" [3] for the postmenopausal women entrusted to our care.

According to Da Silva and coworkers [5] 40% of women are in a postmenopausal state, and 50% to 70% of women report some symptoms of GSM. Symptoms are mild, moderate, or debilitating [6] and impact quality of life, urinary health and control of micturition, pelvic pain disorders, and tissue health and integrity [1]. Women who experience a premature menopause (natural or surgical), or who have had endocrine receptor chemotherapy or radiation therapy to the genital tissue are also at risk for GSM. Therefore, it is important for the clinician to include GSM in their clinical assessment for women, notably when the female patient complains of genital symptoms related to the bladder and vagina, or her sexual function. According to data from the Women's Health Initiative study, although physiologic changes may be present not all women note a complaint in the genitourinary system to their health care provider [6].

Physiology of the genitourinary tract

Estrogen receptors are present in the vagina, vestibule of the vulva, urethra, and trigone of the bladder, and on autonomic and sensory neurons in the vagina and vulva [6]. Testosterone receptors are concentrated in the vulva with fewer in the vagina. Progesterone receptors are found in the vagina and the vulvovaginal epithelial junction [6,7]. Endocrine impact on the genitourinary tract is primarily influenced by estrogen and to a lesser degree by testosterone, dehydroepiandrosterone (DHEA), and progesterone (Box 1).

THE INFLUENCE OF HORMONES ON GENITAL TISSUE HEALTH

During a woman's reproductive years (from puberty until menopause) the urogenital system maintains normal anatomy and physiology through the influence of estrogen. Urogenital hormone receptors in the vagina, vulva, urethra, and trigone of the bladder respond to estrogen stimulation to maintain normal blood flow, tissue thickness, rugae, and elasticity, and epithelial surfaces remain moist. This estrogen-responsive tissue is rich in glycogen, which the normal flora lactobacilli convert to lactic acid. This then maintains an acidic pH of 3.5 to 5.0, maintaining a normal flora to reduce vaginal and urinary system infections [8,9].

As the tissue ages, sclerosis of the microvascular system in addition to loss of estrogen's influence causes the tissue to become thin, fragile with less elasticity, and less of the supportive collagen layers. On the cellular level, the number of parabasal cells increase, and superficial cells are lost [6]. The combination of decreased blood flow through the microvascular system, in addition to the more fragile walls of the vagina cause atrophic cellulitis: cells are degraded and friable.

A hypoestrogenic state results in the fusion of collagen fibers and fragmentation of elastin fibers in vulvovaginal tissue and decreases squamous cells,

> **Box 1: Endocrine influence on the genitourinary tract**
>
> Increase thickness of labia and vulva
>
> Improve collagen, elasticity, and blood flow
>
> Moisturize vaginal mucosa with vaginal and cervical secretions
>
> Increase pubic hair
>
> Balance the vaginal microbiome through influencing vaginal cell glycogen release, thereby lowering vaginal pH to a bacteriostatic level of 3.5 to 4.2
>
> Improve pelvic floor strength and control of neuromuscular component (pudendal nerve mediated for pelvic floor)
>
> Moisturize and thicken the epithelial layers
>
> Enhance suppleness of the vagina, improving the length and width to accommodate sexual activity with additional folds of the rugae
>
> Improve bladder capacity and sensation to pressure, the sphincter's ability to maintain closure
>
> Enhance blood flow for arousal and orgasm to the clitoris and vestibular bulbs (deep in labia minora)
>
> Enhance vaginal sensitivity and tumescence in response to sexual stimulation

resulting in decreased mucosal elasticity and decreased rugae, and narrowing the vagina [10].

Vulvovaginal effects from loss of estrogen include the following [6]:

- Loss of labial and vulval fullness
- Contraction of labia majora and clitoral hood
- Narrowing and stenosis of the introitus
- Loss of elasticity
- Vaginal shortening and narrowing
- Prolapse
- Pelvic floor weakening
- Vaginal epithelium dry and thin with petechiae
- Loss of superficial cells and increase in parabasal cells
- Loss of vaginal rugae
- Inflamed vaginal tissues
- Alkaline pH changes the vaginal microbiome with loss of lactobacilli (vaginal pH >4.5)
- Persistent or recurrent discharge with odor
- Urethral meatal prominence and prolapse with thinning of the urethral epithelium
- Touch perception altered, either hypersensitive or decreased

GENITOURINARY SYNDROME OF MENOPAUSE SIGNS AND SYMPTOMS

The most commonly reported symptoms of GSM are irritation of the vulva, inadequate vaginal lubrication, burning of genital tissue, dysuria, dyspareunia, and vaginal discharge [1]. Signs of GSM include labial atrophy, vaginal dryness, introital stenosis, clitoral atrophy, and phimosis of the prepuce. Severe GSM can cause a friable vaginal wall with the presence of petechiae, ulcerations, tears, hypopigmentation, and bleeding with minimal irritation. "Genitourinary atrophic changes increase the likelihood of trauma, pain, recurrent urinary tract infections, bleeding with or after sex, and absence of sexual activity" [1]. As the symptoms of GSM progress with menopause and lack of estrogen, the genital tissue damage also progresses without effective treatment and intervention [5].

Scavello and colleagues [11] reported that sexual function worsens with advancing menopausal status, and the most frequently reported symptoms are low desire, poor lubrication, and dyspareunia as complications of GSM. Addressing the impact of menopause on sexual intimacy is a component of comprehensive women's health care. Women's sexual function is multifactorial; addressing GSM and aging's impact on relationship intimacy is an important component of comprehensive primary care of women.

PHYSICAL EXAMINATION
The clinician performs a visual and digital examination of the genital tissue, with attention to the pubococcygeus muscle for vaginal wall support, evaluating for adnexal tenderness or fullness with presenting complaints of discomfort, itching, dyspareunia, vaginal discharge, or urinary problems. The vulva are examined for fusion of the labia, presence of ulcers or lesions, discoloration, or signs of genital trauma. Any ulcers or lesions warrant further investigation for cause and if the lesion is pathognomonic of vaginal irritation or pain. The vagina is assessed using the Vaginal Health Index (VHI) (Table 1) as a baseline and during treatment to determine efficacy of therapies. The VHI is an assessment rubric that allows objective determination of the parameters of vaginal health for documentation [12]. Palpation of the vaginal walls can determine presence of pelvic support problems, cystocele or rectocele, and the pelvic examination to determine status of adnexa and periadnexal tissue [13].

USE OF PHARMACOLOGIC AND NUTRACEUTICAL AGENTS
When deciding on agents to offer the patient with GSM, it is advisable for the clinician to determine impact of the atrophy and consider physiology of the urogenital tissue. If she reports dryness being the primary issue, moisturizers or lubricants are used.

First-line treatment
Patients who have mild symptoms from GSM should be informed of available options regarding use of vaginal moisturizers and lubricants. This includes guidance of using a pH-balanced, low-osmolality option. Women with mild GSM often find this therapy is adequate to enhance comfort [1]. Lubricants differ from moisturizers; lubricants are not absorbed by the genital epithelia and are designed to reduce friction-related irritation. Moisturizers are

| | | Fluid secretion, | | | |
Score	Overall elasticity	type and consistency	pH	Epithelial mucosa	Moisture
1	None	None	6.1	Petechiae noted before contact	None, mucosa inflamed
2	Poor	Scant, thin yellow	5.6–6.0	Bleeds with light contact	None, mucosa not inflamed
3	Fair	Superficial, thin white	5.1–5.5	Bleeds with scraping	Minimal
4	Good	Moderate, thin white	4.7–5.0	Not friable, thin mucosa	Moderate
5	Excellent	Normal (white flocculent)	<4.6	Not friable, normal mucosa	Normal

Table 1
Vaginal Health Index

(From Bachmann G. Urogenital aging: an old problem newly recognized. Maturitas. 1995;22 Suppl:S1-S5. https://doi.org/10.1016/0378-51229500956-6) with permission)

hydrophobic; are absorbed by the genital epithelia; can address pH balance; and because moisturizers are bioadhesive, they mimic the vaginal secretions [5]. Women are recommended to use lubricants for sexual activity as needed, and moisturizers on a routine basis independent of sexual activity. There are several products available that work as moisturizer and lubricant. Hyaluronic acid has been used to alleviate vaginal dryness; although studies are small it may be helpful to treat GSM [14–16]. Hyaluronic acid is an essential ingredient in topical hydrating and lubricating gels; it is a naturally occurring polysaccharide that can increase hydration of cells and improve symptoms of vaginal atrophy.

The efficacy of these over-the-counter agents is dependent on mechanics and tissue response. Glycol-based moisturizers and lubricants can be irritating to the nontreated (low estrogen) postmenopausal vagina, causing irritation and pain. High-osmolarity (concentration of solid per fluid) products can cause irritation and cytotoxicity; the World Health Organization recommends the osmolality (fluid to electrolyte concentration, similar physiologically to osmolarity within tissue) of a personal lubricant not exceed 380 mOsm/kg to avoid epithelial damage or cytotoxicity [14]. The more viscous the agent, the more irritation may occur: a watery agent is less irritating than a thicker, gellike agent. Moisturizers rehydrate the tissue, and efficacy is based on osmolality and pH [17]. Moisturizers based with beeswax should be avoided by women with allergies to bees, and coconut oil is an irritant if the woman is also allergic to tree nuts. "Vaginal products and their ingredients affect bacteria growth and viability in vitro, conclusive literature on effects in vivo is lacking" [18]. In addition to recommending treatment options (moisturizers or vaginal estrogen) if the primary complaint is irritation the patient should be cautioned to avoid irritants to the tissue. Soaps, perfumes, douche, petroleum-based products, feminine hygiene products, and excessive cleaning may disrupt the pH balance [13]. Vaginal irritants to avoid include [5]

- Soaps
- Perfumes
- Douche
- Petroleum-based products
- Feminine hygiene products
- Excessive cleaning that disrupts the natural microbiome
- Glycol-based lubricants
- Potential allergen triggers
- Smoking use: this increases metabolism of estrogen, leading to atrophic changes

If your patient reports more symptoms than occasional dryness, pharmaceutical agents may then be considered. Recall from the discussion about physiology that estrogen α receptors in the vagina are primarily active postmenopause. Testosterone receptors are concentrated in the vulva, less in vaginal tissue; progesterone receptors are in the vagina and the vulvovaginal epithelial junction [6]. When using a topical hormone treatment, where the topical agent is applied determines absorption and efficacy. The vaginal estrogen creams (estradiol, estrone sulfate) are designed to use a suspending agent with the active hormone to trigger hormone receptors and the suspending agent to provide some moisture. For those women with more advanced atrophy, noted with lower scores on the VHI, NAMS has recommended first-line treatment of vaginal estrogen therapy [1] at a low dose and until efficacy is achieved. Da Silva and colleagues [5] reported that most studies indicate significant improvement of dyspareunia when vaginal estrogen is used in addition to lubricants. Specific options of creams, vaginal inserts, and systemic therapies can be reviewed with the patient on a case-by-case basis, incorporating patient preference and individualized risk.

Vaginal therapies
Vaginal therapy is the first-line pharmacologic treatment recommended by NAMS [1] and the International Menopause Society for GSM [14].

Vaginal estradiol
The dosage of vaginal estradiol is low. An advantage for use is that there is minimal systemic absorption; the greatest rise in serum levels actually occurs during the first 24 to 72 hours of use and does not remain increased [5]. Serum levels of hormones in the vaginal estrogen user do not achieve the level of postmenopausal androgen release from adrenal source; however, there are limited studies comparing products in a broad population. The reader is encouraged to recollect from the discussion about physiology that there are estrone (E1), estradiol (E2), estriol (E3), testosterone, progesterone, and DHEA receptors in the genitourinary system. With vaginal estrogens, estrone is minimally

absorbed, estriol is minimally effective at receptor sites (10%), and the vaginal hormone receptors for α-estradiol are most effectively treated with topical estradiol agents (ring, tablet, cream) [5,18] because the primary estrogen receptor in genital tissue responds to estradiol. If you have a patient with previous estradiol receptor–positive cancer (eg, the breast) using vaginal estrogen (E1, E2, or E3) should be discussed with her oncology medical care team; although there is minimal systemic absorption of vaginal estrogens, and benefits of short-term therapy to treat GSM may outweigh potential risk, there are limited research studies about using vaginal estrogen agents post-estrogen-dependent cancer treatment. Systemic absorption of estrogen may be a concern regarding use of vaginal estrogen therapy, so careful consideration regarding its use is recommended.

Postmenopausal women who are taking hormone therapy systemically (oral or transdermal) to treat vasomotor symptoms of menopause may still experience symptoms of GSM. Studies [5] have indicated these women benefit from additional vaginal estrogen use because 30% of women on systemic hormone therapy report vaginal dryness and dyspareunia.

Prasterone, a vaginal insert in a synthetic form of DHEA, yields the metabolites estradiol and testosterone. Recall from the physiology review that there are testosterone receptors in external genitalia, and estradiol receptors in the vagina, trigone of the bladder, and labia minora. Daily use of prasterone for women with moderate to severe dyspareunia often yields a significant reduction in subjective symptoms, improved superficial and parabasal cells, and an improvement in vaginal pH [15,19]. Prasterone also improves the VHI objectively [5]. Prasterone has not been shown to increase serum levels of estradiol or testosterone, but further studies need to be performed in women with a history of hormonal cancers [5].

Alternative treatments include selective estrogen receptor modulators, such as ospemifene [14], a tissue-selective estrogen complex, and herbal therapies. There are limited studies on the use of herbal therapies to treat GSM; oral and topical agents are available widely and anecdotal studies report some improvement in symptoms, although it is not clear whether this is caused by additional moisture (with topical agents) or a shift in the vaginal pH. It is best to assess what over-the-counter agents have been used by your patient to determine if her symptoms of pain or irritation are caused by GSM or by the nutraceutical (herbal, over-the-counter) agent she is using.

Ospemifene is a selective estrogen receptor modulator, indicated for severe dyspareunia. Considered an alternative to vaginal estrogen therapy, it has been shown to have a beneficial effect on vaginal dryness, decreasing the vaginal pH, reducing parabasal cells, and increasing superficial cells [5,14]. Ospemifene is the only oral agent approved by the Food and Drug Administration (FDA) for nonhormonal treatment of GSM because it has been found to address vaginal stenosis, mucosal moisture, and vaginal epithelial thickness and pH [5]. Use of this agent in women with moderate to severe GSM improved vaginal comfort and urinary symptoms.

Full prescribing information for the previously mentioned hormone thera-pies is beyond the scope of this article. The reader is encouraged to review full prescribing details for specific agents.

Compounded hormonal preparations have not received FDA approval, and as such are not recommended for use [1]. Compounded agents are available through specialty pharmacies and through online pharmaceutical supply sour-ces. Estriol vaginal cream is also not approved by the FDA, but is widely avail-able outside of the United States for treatment of GSM [14,15]. Estriol is minimally effective (10%) at the estrogen receptor sites in the vagina and studies of efficacy and long-term benefits versus risk are still pending in the United States [1]. Estriol does not convert to estradiol in vivo or in vitro, and as such there is little systemic absorption [5].

Other medication influences on genital tissue

A comprehensive evaluation of the GSM patient's presenting complaint may uncover contributing factors for vaginal dryness; lack of sexual response (arousal or orgasm); poor libido; or bladder complaints of pain, incontinence, or frequency. Many medications and over-the-counter supplements influence the genital tissue. It may require adjustment of other medications (eg, antihis-tamines, antihypertensives, neuromuscular agents) to improve vaginal mois-ture or tissue response to efforts. Adjustments may include timing of the medication administration, alternative therapies, or stopping use if not therapeutic.

Vaginal dryness can occur secondary to use of antihistamines, or anticholin-ergic agents for overactive bladder. Some diuretics may cause vaginal dryness. If in review of all medications used, a potential side effect is mouth dryness then the culprit for a new vaginal complaint may be the agent causing mucous membrane dryness.

Agents used to control hypertension are often not sexually friendly, although some antihypertensives are less likely to cause anorgasmia. Helping with timing of medications used may help the patient be more compliant with taking her blood pressure medications and still maintain a sexual response that she de-sires. As an example, if sexual activity is primarily in the evening, taking her medications just before sex may diminish the poor response to genital stimula-tion, because peak effect of most antihypertensives is 6 to 10 hours after administration.

Medications to treat overactive bladder or urinary incontinence can diminish lubrication to genital tissue. If an agent has a possible side effect of bladder spasms, this can be a cause for genital pain with sexual activity. Modifying when the agent is taken (holding dose until after sex) may reduce dyspareunia that is triggered by the use of the anticholinergic agent (eg, tolterodine).

EXERCISES TO IMPROVE MUSCLE TONE AND BLOOD FLOW

A low-cost and effective recommendation to enhance blood flow and muscle tone of the pelvis is through the use of Kegel exercises. The woman needs instruction to begin by focusing on the pubococcygeus muscle, and tightening the muscle that surrounds the vagina, urethra, and rectum. Explaining that the tissue deep within the pelvic sling is exercised with Kegels to improve tone, enhance the ability of the organs to stay aligned, and maintain tissue may be helpful. It is recommended that the clinician assess the muscle tone of the vagina by performing a digital vaginal examination and then with fingers still inserted asking the woman to Kegel, or tighten, the vaginal walls (Table 2). In this way the clinician can ascertain that the muscle is targeted correctly by the patient and responding to her efforts.

Another recommendation is to have women do their "Kegels" throughout the day. When I discuss treatment options for waning libido, I recommend that women perform Kegels daily, but also add the biofeedback technique of having the woman visualize her partner (even looking at them or their picture) while doing her Kegel to improve the genital response of arousal (engorgement of the genital tissue) that is then associated with her partner.

Referral to be evaluated for treatment with a physical therapist specializing in pelvic floor concerns can also be beneficial to patients to help address urinary symptoms, such as incontinence or retention, severe dyspareunia, and pelvic prolapse [14]. Pelvic floor physical therapy may not be widely available to many women, dependent on geography and insurance coverage. Many women benefit, however, from therapy targeting the pelvic muscles and genital tissue response and physical therapy should be considered as a viable treatment option when first-line therapies do not address concerns of pain, bladder control, or vaginal tone.

SURGICAL INTERVENTIONS

Considering surgical interventions (referral to a genitourinary surgeon) may include fractional laser therapy and transcutaneous temperature-controlled radiofrequency with external and internal treatments to improve vaginal dryness, vulvovaginal laxity, and dyspareunia [10]. Light amplification by stimulated emission of radiation (laser) techniques include the use of

Table 2
Assessment of vaginal tone with Kegel/tightening the pubococcygeus muscle

Value	Findings
1	Patient unable to target muscle, weak flick of the muscle, little determination that there has been any change in vaginal tone.
2	Mild squeeze of the vagina in response to Kegel, little change to bladder position (cystocele persists).
3	Vagina wall snugs lower half around examiner's fingers, bladder aligns midway if cystocele present. Visible change at introitus with movement of perineum and labia.
4	Vagina wall firm muscle tone that is maintained, correction of cystocele or rectocele. Vaginal introitus tightens.

nonablative photothermal erbium:YAG laser and carbon dioxide laser. Through thermomodulation, these laser technologies restore the vaginal epithelium to that of a premenopausal woman by causing collagen remodeling, neovascularization, vasodilation, and the formation of elastin [5]. Several small studies have shown that fractional carbon dioxide laser therapy can restore the vaginal epithelium to a state similar to the premenopausal state, increase the amounts of lactobacillus and other premenopausal flora, and improve the VHI score and subjective symptoms of GSM, including lower urinary tract symptoms [14]. The use of the erbium:YAG laser has been shown to improve symptoms of GSM and stress urinary incontinence. These therapies are being studied further, and routine use of laser therapy to treat GSM has yet to achieve FDA approval; in 2018 the FDA issued a statement that safety and efficacy studies were still pending on vaginal rejuvenation treatments with laser [5].

FOLLOW-UP

Deciding on when a patient should follow up for evaluation for the treatment of GSM is dependent on degree of impact. It is recommended that your assessment continue to determine therapy efficacy. Performing a VHI at follow-up visits may help with determining if a dose adjustment is required. Vaginal hormone therapy may be adjusted to a maintenance dose once moisture and improved comfort are attained. If lesions are present, they should be assessed further. Any undiagnosed vaginal bleeding warrants thorough evaluation and possible referral to a gynecology nurse practitioner or physician to rule out neoplasm [13]. Routine gynecologic health screenings (eg, pap smear, pelvic examination) should continue as part of comprehensive standard women's health.

Billing and coding

GSM does not have a specific International Classification of Diseases (ICD)-10 code at this time. The billable ICD-10 code used is the same as one used for postmenopausal atrophic vaginitis (N95.1). This ICD-10 code is also used for menopausal and female climacteric states.

PATIENT CASE SCENARIO AND DISCUSSION

Urinary signs and symptoms

Patricia (62 years old) presents to the office with a complaint of "another bladder infection" with frequency, some mild incontinence when bladder full, and discomfort when touching the urethral meatus. Patricia is postmenopausal (spontaneous) by 8 years, and her problem list includes diet-controlled diabetes (hemoglobin A_{1C} of 6.4), a body mass index of 32, and osteoarthritis of bilateral knees. Medications include lisinopril 5 mg, meloxicam 7.5 mg, multivitamin, and calcium with D_3, and she maintains normal physical activity. She is sexually active with her spouse of 38 years and practices postcoital prevention measures (voiding, care with wiping, using a nonirritating lubricant). She was on a combination (estradiol-progestin) hormone therapy for 5 years to treat vasomotor symptoms, stopping this 3 years ago. Patricia has been to the office four times in the previous 14 months with the same complaints. Urinalysis via point-of-care testing indicates white blood cells small, no nitrites, small amount of blood. On examination the labia minora and majora are partially fused, pale, thin but nonsclerotic tissue, urethral meatus protrudes slightly and is also pale. The VHI score today is 13: elasticity is rated at 2, fluid secretion 3, pH is 6.0 (score 2), epithelium is scored at 4, and moisture rates a 2. This is improved over her VHI of 8 months prior (score 8) when she reported genital dryness and began to use coconut oil as a moisturizer and lubricant to the genitalia (vulva and vagina), and began doing Kegels 30 to 50 times daily. There is a mild cystocele present, and Kegel muscle strength is rated 3 out of 4 (snug pubococcygeus muscle around examiner's gloved fingers, which brings the bladder up into a normal midline position). Adnexa are small and mobile, uterus midline, with normal size, shape, and mobility for a G1P1 female. Urine specimen from today will be sent to the laboratory for microbiology testing (to rule out *Escherichia coli* infection because of pyuria), and to cytology (sending some urine in a liquid medium for evaluation of the hematuria to screen for urothelial neoplasm). Patricia and I then began a dialogue about GSM and that her evaluation today in the office indicated it was not likely an infection but may be caused by the hypoestrogenic genital tissue. After discussing benefits, expected side effects, and options for using vaginal estradiol therapy Patricia opted to use a vaginal estradiol 2-mg ring. She was concerned that the cream may be too messy and wanted the benefit of the modified pessary action of the ring. We also discussed that her partner may feel the ring, but it would not cause him any discomfort, and if the ring slipped during the 90-day use, how to clean and replace the device. Patricia agreed to return to the office in 4 to 6 months for a recheck and was asked to monitor her symptoms of vaginal dryness, urinary complaints, and to notify me of any vaginal bleeding. The urinalysis was reported normal 24 hours after her visit, and cytology report was "no urothelial cell malignancy detected" per pathology 1 week later. Patricia returned to the office for her routine wellness examination 5 months after her visit for urinary complaints. She reported that she no longer felt vaginal dryness, only using a small amount of coconut oil with sexual activity to enhance her response. She had no occurrences of urinary frequency or urethral meatus tenderness in the past 5 months and noted improved control of her bladder. VHI score was rated at 18 (elasticity 4, fluid secretion 3, vaginal pH 5.1 now rated 3, epithelial cells 4, and moisture 4). She was pleased with the therapy results; found the replacement after 90 days to be easy to perform; and the repeat point-of-care testing of her urine clean catch in the office was normal with no hematuria, white cells, or nitrites. We agreed to revisit the vaginal estradiol therapy annually at her wellness examinations, and she was reminded to advise me of any vaginal bleeding or abnormal discharge.

SUMMARY

GSM is a common disorder of menopause, experienced to some degree by more than 80% of menopausal women. Pharmacologic and lifestyle changes can help maintain function and reduce symptoms associated with this disorder. The primary care provider of a menopausal woman is able to assess the impact of endocrine loss on genital tissue and sexual function and begin to address the symptoms. Sexual function in women is multifactorial and addressing vaginal lubrication and the presence of pain or discomfort may help the menopausal patient maintain their relationship intimacy. In contrast to other symptoms associated with menopause (eg, vasomotor symptoms, which diminish over time) genitourinary syndrome is likely to be progressive in severity and symptoms without intervention. It rarely resolves without intervention.

Disclosure

None to report.

References

[1] North American Menopause Society (NAMS). NAMS Position Statement: the 2020 genitourinary syndrome of menopause position statement of the North American Menopause Society. Menopause 2020;27(9):976–92; https://doi.org/10.1097/GME.000000 000000001609.

[2] Alvasi S, Gava G, Orsili I, et al. Vaginal health in menopausal women medicine. Medicina 2019;55(9):615. Available at: www.mdpi.com/journal/medicina.

[3] Angelou K, Grigoriadis T, Diakosavvas M, et al. The genitourinary syndrome of menopause: an overview of the recent data. Cureus 2020;12(4):e7586; https://doi.org/10.7759/cureus.7586.

[4] Portman DJ, Gass ML. Vulvovaginal Atrophy Terminology Consensus Conference Panel. Genitourinary syndrome of menopause: new terminology for vulvovaginal atrophy from the International Society for the Study of Women's Sexual Health and the North American Menopause Society. Climacteric 2014;17:557–63.

[5] Da Silva AS, Baines G, Araklitis G, et al. Modern management of genitourinary syndrome of menopause. Fac Rev 2021;10(25); https://doi.org/10.12703/r/10-25.

[6] Farrell E. Genitourinary syndrome of menopause. Aust Fam Pract 2017;46(7):481–4.

[7] Traish A, Vignozzi L, Simon J, et al. Role of androgens in female genitourinary tissue structure and function: implications in the genitourinary syndrome of menopause. Sex Med Rev 2018;6(4):558–71.

[8] Bleibel, B. & Nguyen, H. 2021 Vaginal Atrophy StatPearls [internet]. PMID: 32644723.

[9] White BA, Harrison JR, Mehlmann LM. Endocrine and reproductive physiology: Mosby physiology Series. 5th Edition. St. Louis, MO: Elsevier; 2019.

[10] Flores, S.A., Hall, C.A. Atrophic Vaginitis. 2021. StatPearls.

[11] Scavello I, Maseroli E, DI Stasi V, et al. Sexual health in menopause. Medicina 2019;55:559; https://doi.org/10.3390/medicina55090559/. www.mdpi.com/journal/medicina.

[12] Bachmann G. Urogenital ageing: an old problem newly recognized. Maturitas 1995;(Supple. 1):S1–5.

[13] Phillips NA, Bachmann GA. Genitourinary syndrome of menopause: common problem, effective treatments. Cleveland Clin J Med 2018;85(5):390–8.

[14] Kagan R, Kellogg-Spadt S, Parish SJ. Practical treatment considerations in the management of genitourinary syndrome of menopause. Drugs & Aging 2019;36:897–908; https://doi.org/10.1007/s40266-019-00700-w.

[15] Shim S, Park K-M, Chung Y-J, et al. Updates on therapeutic alternatives for genitourinary syndrome of menopause: hormonal and non-hormonal managements. J Menopausal Med 2021;27:1–7; https://doi.org/10.6118/jmm.20034.

[16] Ford L. A mixed methods analysis of the concept of female sexual health. [Doctoral Dissertation, Western Michigan University; 2007.

[17] Edwards D, Panay N. Treating vulvovaginal atrophy/genitourinary syndrome of menopause: how important is vaginal lubricant and moisturizer composition? Climacteric 2016;19(2):151–61.

[18] Hung KJ, Hudson PL, Bergerat A, et al. Effect of commercial vaginal products on the growth of uropathogenic and commensal vaginal bacteria. Scientific Rep 2020;10:7625; https://doi.org/10.1038/s4598-020-63652-x.

[19] AMAG Pharmaceuticals, Inc. Intrarosa Full Prescribing Information. 2016. Available at: www.intrarosa.com.

Postpartum Depression
Updates in Evaluation and Care

Katharine Green, PhD, CNM[a],*,
Maud Low, PhD, RNC, CLNC[a]

[a]Elaine Marieb College of Nursing, University of Massachuasetts AmherstSkinner Hall, 651 North Pleasant St., Amherst, MA 01003, USA

Keywords

- Postpartum depression • PPD evaluation and care • Peripartum depression

Key points

- Postpartum depression incidence is increasing and should be screened for at antepartum, postpartum, and pediatric visits.
- Therapeutic counseling should be used as a first step in all peripartal people who are at risk of postpartum depression.
- Good informal social support may help prevent and may decrease the symptoms of postpartum depression.
- There are multiple treatment modalities available for postpartum depression, including counseling, medication, social support, repeated transcranial magnetic stimulation, and electroconvulsive therapy.
- The rare complication of postpartum psychosis is a medical emergency and requires emergent hospitalization and treatment.

INTRODUCTION

Postpartum depression (PPD) is a relatively common depressive disorder that occurs after the delivery of a baby. Previously thought to have an onset only after delivery, postpartum depression is now considered to be a form of peripartal depression, as approximately half of cases have an onset of affective symptoms during pregnancy [1]. PPD is a major depressive disorder (MDD) that can be managed with nonpharmaceutical therapeutic care in less serious cases, but often requires more extensive treatment [1,2].

*Corresponding author. Elaine Marieb College of Nursing, University of Massachuasetts AmherstSkinner Hall, 651 N. Pleasant St. Amherst, MA 01003, USA E-mail address: kgreen@nursing.umass.edu

https://doi.org/10.1016/j.yfpn.2021.12.008
2589-420X/22/© 2021 Elsevier Inc. All rights reserved.

Peripartum depression is defined by the American Psychiatric Association as depression that occurs during pregnancy or after delivery and includes symptoms of sadness, changes in energy that may include reduced capacity for pleasure, sleep issues, appetite changes, and anxiety [1–3]. Patients may exhibit loss of interest, reduced capacity to think clearly, and an inability to concentrate. (PPP), a severe form of PPD, is a condition that may include suicidal or infanticidal ideation and requires emergency psychiatric evaluation [2]. Symptoms of PPD may begin as early as the third trimester of pregnancy or may start as late as 4 weeks to 1 year postpartum [2–4].

Peripartal depression is a common complication of childbearing. Although estimates vary, it is suspected that as many as 1 in 7 childbearing women may be affected, and recent work suggests that the incidence may be increasing [1–6]. Although part of the increase is suspected to be related to increased awareness and diagnosis, there was a 30% increase in peripartal depression between 2014 and 2018, possibly related to income inequality, women's long working hours, older maternal age, and decreased social connections [6,7]. The childbearing parent, newborn, and entire family unit are likely to suffer long-term effects from perinatal depression [1–5].

Estimates of the incidence of PPD vary greatly, from 6% to 20% of childbearing women [3,7]. Although there is regional variation, an increased incidence in PPD exceeding 20% has been found in women who were adolescents, smokers, those who had a history of intimate partner violence or a prior history of depression, those who suffered the death of an infant, or those who were of Native American or Alaskan Native heritage [8]. Half of the depressive episodes in the peripartal period are diagnosed during pregnancy, and 50% of cases are diagnosed up to 1 year postpartum [3,8].

TYPES OF DEPRESSION POSTPARTUM

PPD, the subset of peripartum depression that occurs after delivery, has been divided into categories, each of which has its own incidence, risk factors, prognosis, and outcomes. These categories include "baby blues," PPD, and PPP.

Baby blues

"Baby blues" is a common short-lived phenomenon lasting only several days within the first 2 weeks following birth. Characterized by sadness or moodiness, "baby blues" do not require treatment, resolve spontaneously, and are estimated to be experienced by up to 70% of childbearing women [4]. "Baby blues" are not PPD, as they are related to the changes in hormonal levels, fatigue, and relationship changes. "Baby blues" occur in 39% to -85% of women, typically improve spontaneously within 3 to 5 days, and require no treatment [9–11].

Postpartum depression

PPD, a subset of peripartal depression, typically occurs later after the birth of a baby and may have some of the same symptoms as postpartum blues. However, PPD lasts longer than 2 weeks and is likely to require treatment [2].

Although the underlying cause is not known, PPD may be related to a sudden drop in estrogen and progesterone or thyroid hormones following delivery, fatigue from labor and delivery, sleep disruption, or relationship changes. Changes in home life, work, unscheduled time, unrealistic expectations, and being overwhelmed may also be related. PPD is associated with poor bonding with the newborn and later disruptions in cognitive, emotional, and physical development in children. PPD is disruptive to the patient and their family and is a serious illness [11].

Symptoms of PPD are similar to other MDD and include sadness, hopelessness, restlessness, moodiness, low energy, and difficulty focusing or with memory (Table 1). The postpartum person may have multiple other symptoms that do not dissipate spontaneously, and the patient or family members may notice symptoms worsening [2,4,10,11].

Postpartum psychosis

PPP is rare, occurring in 1 to 4 out of 1000 postpartum women, and occurs within the first 2 days to 4 weeks postpartum [11,12]. In addition to other symptoms of PPD, people with PPP may suffer from hallucinations, paranoia, agitation, reckless behavior, confusion, and very rapid mood swings. The patient, the newborn, and other children are at high risk of injury or death, as the patient may become suicidal or consider infanticide [4,11]. Frequently related to a past personal or family history of bipolar disorder, PPP is considered a medical emergency and is frightening for the patient and their family.

Women who have the preexisting mental health conditions, such as bipolar disorder or schizoaffective disorder, are at higher risk of PPP [13,14]. Furthermore, bipolar disorder may emerge during pregnancy in birthing parents who

Table 1
Symptoms of postpartum depression

Common symptoms of PPD	Less common symptoms of PPD
Sadness	Disconnection with activities once enjoyed
Hopelessness	Difficulty with memory
Restlessness	Thoughts of harming self or baby
Crying	Stomach and bowel issues
Moodiness	Headaches vague pains or aching
Low energy	Anxiety
Difficulty focusing	Unable to relax
Feeling overwhelmed	Chest pain
Feeling disconnected from baby	Sleep too much or too little
Overeating or undereating	Feeling worthless
Disconnection from family and friends	
Feeling like inadequate parent	
Guilt	

Data from Beck CT. A checklist to identify women at risk for developing postpartum depression.J Obstet Gynecol Neonatal Nurs. 1998;27(1):39-46 have a personal or family history of mood disorders [4]. Patients may suffer from severe sadness, high energy, elevated mood, rapid speech, poor judgment, minimal sleep, and hallucinations or delusions [4].

HISTORY

Mental health disorders attributable to or coinciding with events in female lives have been recognized for centuries. From nearly 4000 years ago when Romans diagnosed hysteria, from the root word hystera, or uterus, PPD was suggested to be a type of female mental illness through "puerperal melancholia." In the 1800s, women were vulnerable to mental illnesses related to childbearing [15,16]. Treatments over the ages included ice baths, restraint, bleeding, purging, food, rest, and institutionalization of affected women. During the early part of the twentieth century, motherhood was extolled, and little mention was made of PPD or other negative emotions that might be related to childbearing [16].

However, in the 1950s, some articles in the popular press had started to mention PPD, although it went against the narrative of joyous motherhood embraced in the first part of the century for white middle-class women, the societal standard to which all women were compared at the time [17]. By the mid-1980s, PPD was recognized as a poorly understood distinct illness that not only affected the postpartum mother but also negatively affected the newborn and the family constellation [10,15]. Little screening was done for PPD [10,15].

At the end of the twentieth century, researchers had recognized the need for screening and intervention for PPD. Several models were developed to evaluate postpartum women for PPD. Two widely used scales developed for this purpose were the Beck Postpartum Depression Screening Scale and the Edinburgh Postnatal Depression Scale, both of which helped care providers evaluate the need for intervention in postpartum patients [10,12].

Interest in PPD has accelerated since the turn of the century. The US Preventative Services Taskforce (USPSTF) updated its screening recommendations for depression in adults to include screening of pregnant and postpartum women and in 2019 recommended counseling intervention for all pregnant or postpartum women who showed symptoms of depression [5].

EFFECTS OF THE CORONAVIRUS DISEASE 2019 PANDEMIC ON POSTPARTUM DEPRESSION

It is estimated that only about 50% of women who had PPD were diagnosed as such before the coronavirus disease 2019 (COVID-19) pandemic [18]. The Kaiser Family Foundation has reported that the baseline rate of depression and anxiety in the adult population of the United States has increased precipitously since the onset of the COVID-19 pandemic in early 2020 [19]. Although approximately 11% of the population reported symptoms of anxiety and depression in a survey done in the first half of 2019, the Kaiser survey showed an incidence of anxiety and depression of approximately 41% in 2021 [19].

Because a prior history of depression and anxiety is associated with PPD, it is unsurprising that anxiety and depression in pregnant and postpartum women may also have become more prevalent during the pandemic. Of concern, the continuing isolation from friends and family that the COVID-19 pandemic has required could further increased PPD.

DIAGNOSIS

Diagnosis of PPD is made via the persistence of troubling depressive symptoms that affect thinking, mood and emotions, and daily activities, including care of self and others, sleep, eating, and work, for 2 weeks or longer [2]. Diagnosis of PPD is dependent on the presence of 5 or more signs and symptoms that last more than 2 weeks (Box 1) [20]. As with other diagnoses, PPD should be considered against the individual's complete evaluation, which should include thyroid levels and a complete physical examination.

RISK FACTORS

Risk factors for PPD may include a past history of depression, anxiety, or PPD in the patient or their family, current life stress, a history of sexual or physical abuse, pregnancy complications including preterm or traumatic deliveries, or

---

Box 1: Postpartum depression symptoms from *Diagnostic and Statistical Manual of Mental Disorders* (Fifth Edition)

Feeling of depression most of day, most days for greater than 2 weeks

Decreased pleasure or interest in usual pastimes for greater than 2 weeks

Eating more or less than usual; gaining or losing weight, appetite changes

Sleeping more or less than usual

Agitation, fidgeting, slower movements, or slower talking than usual

Feeling tired or run down most of day, most days for greater than 2 weeks

Difficulty concentrating

Memory loss

Difficulty making decisions

Feeling worthless, guilty, or overwhelmed

Thoughts of death or suicide or current suicidal ideation

Inability to take care of self (hygiene, meals, food)

Inability to take care of baby or feeling detached from baby

Detachment from family and friends

Inability to work, study, or maintain household

Inability to problem solve or cope with problems

Data from American Psychiatric Association. Diagnostic and statistical manual of mental disorders (DSM-5). 5th ed. Washington DC; American Psychiatric Associatsww2ion, 2013.

difficulty during labor [1–3,21,22]. Young maternal age, poor or limited social support, low economic status, substance use disorder, and unplanned pregnancy may also be risk factors [2,3,22,23]. Although most women experience some stress during pregnancy, there is evidence that black and Hispanic women, particularly those experiencing relational and financial stress, and Asian/Pacific Islander women experiencing high levels of physical stress have higher rates of PPD [18,21]. Impoverished women have rates of PPD that are nearly double those of the general population of childbearing women [22].

SCREENING TOOLS

Although there have been several tools developed to assist in screening for PPD, two are commonly used. The Beck Postpartum Depression Screening Scale is based on risk factors for PPD and is designed to be used as a tool that promotes discussion between a patient and their provider [8]. Beck's scale helps patients, and their providers, consider specific risk factors for PPD in the context of length of time symptoms have occurred (Box 2) [8]. In the Beck screening tool, although a higher score indicates greater risk of PPD, it is not diagnostic. Furthermore, Beck recommended the continued use of the tool to screen throughout the first year of the infant's life, so that women with later-onset PPD could be screened in for further workup [8].

The Edinburgh Postnatal Depression Scale is a shorter, 10-question screening tool that can be completed in approximately 5 minutes by patients or providers [11,18,19]. Although there are no universally accepted cutoff markers diagnostic for depression in this scale, a score of greater than 12 is frequently considered to be indicative of probable PPD and requires further patient evaluation [11,18,19,24].

A 2018 study showed that approximately 80% of women were screened during pregnancy, and 87% were screen postpartum for risk factors related to PPD

Box 2: Primary screening topics in the Beck Postpartum Depression Scale

Antenatal depression

Antenatal anxiety

History of previous depression

Lack of social support

Marital/partner relationship dissatisfaction

Life stress (major life changes, family or partner issues, financial issues, death in family)

Childcare issues

"Baby blues"

Data from: Beck CT. A checklist to identify women at risk for developing postpartum depression. J Obstet Gynecol Neonatal Nurs. 1998; 27(1):39-46

[15]. However, there is some evidence that screening for PPD has significantly declined during the COVID-19 pandemic. As the need to curtail face-to-face visits to protect healthy patients and health care workers increased, the in-person visit schedule for pregnant and postpartum people has significantly decreased, and screening opportunities have lessened [18].

PREVENTION

Little is known about prevention of PPD. The American College of Obstetricians and Gynecologists recommends early screening for all postpartum patients [23]. The USPTF recommends counseling for those at risk for depression and anxiety during pregnancy, as evidence supports moderate beneficial effects for this group [5].

Exercise and diet

There is limited information on the utility of exercise, dietary changes or supplements, or education as preventives of PPD [2]. Although there are recommendations encouraging regular exercise, low-quality evidence and limited studies on exercise and PPD have found modest benefits, although other work has found no benefit [25,26]. High dropout rates among participants in these studies may speak to the difficulty new mothers have with time management owing to disrupted sleep schedules and multiple role demands [25].

Dietary supplements are currently being reviewed in the prevention of peripartum depression by the USPSTF, although recommendations are not yet available [2]. There is exploratory work on the use of vitamin D and selenium as dietary supplements that may have the potential to prevent PPD [27]. Other dietary areas of exploration in prevention of PPD may include combination dietary supplements, or tryptophan, tyrosine, fish oil supplementation, vitamin D, calcium, selenium, blueberries, or combination dietary supplements [27]. Although evidence remains elusive, there may be some role for dietary supplements or hormones in the future.

Social support

There is good evidence that adequate social support is strongly protective against PPD in diverse populations. Informal support from families and friends is instrumental in the postpartum period, particularly for first-time parents, and families should be coached to help with housework, emotional support, and childcare throughout the first year. Partners should be coached to encourage good nutrition and exercise, as well as support women in gaining regular time for themselves [28,29].

In summary, preventative strategies include screening for PPD and referrals for counseling from care providers and the promotion of good social support for all postpartum women. During a time of pandemic, when social interaction outside of a family circle is difficult, it is especially important that all care providers should assess the postpartum patient's mood and affect during all interactions, including during pediatric visits through the first year of the newborn's life. Providers must be prepared to discuss concerning findings and take appropriate action.

Web-based prevention

A newer approach to the prevention of PPD in women at risk for the disorder is the use of Web-based cognitive behavioral therapy (WCBT) emphasizing emotional regulation and self-compassion. Some early explorations of this method in PPD suggest that WCBT shows significant improvement in intervention groups in the short term, particularly when guided by a therapist or therapeutic group of health care providers [30,31]. Further study may elucidate increased applicability of this technique to women with active PPD, particularly with the increased use of teletherapy during the pandemic.

TREATMENT OF POSTPARTUM DEPRESSION

Lifestyle changes

Several lifestyle changes are recommended for those diagnosed with PPD [2]. Instituting or reinstating social support from the patient's own network or support groups for new parents may be helpful. After the initial recovery from delivery, maintaining good nutrition and starting moderate exercise may also be useful. Increasing sleep times when the baby sleeps may mitigate the fatigue of new parents, and time for the new parent to go out or see friends may contribute to recovery [4].

Barriers to care include scarcity of resources and supports for the postpartum patient, even under the best of circumstances. Furthermore, patients with PPD and their families may not feel comfortable reaching out to others for support because of the stigma of mental illness, which may worsen their situation.

Worsening or severe cases of PPD and PPP require more intense treatment. All health care providers should be aware of current treatments, including psychotherapy, medications, homeopathy, transcranial magnetic stimulation, electroconvulsive therapy (ECT), and supplements and hormones.

Psychotherapy

Although there has been some controversy about the efficacy of psychotherapy with a mental health care provider in the treatment of PPD, it is now widely recommended as both initial and adjunct treatment [5,31–34]. Counseling appears to be effective with or without medications in diminishing depressive symptoms for at least the first 12 weeks postpartum, whether in person or via telehealth [35]. Cognitive behavioral therapy has been shown to be efficacious in treating PPD up to 6 months postpartum [30,31,36].

Psychotherapeutic treatments tend to suffer from high dropout rates among patients with PPD. Individuals with PPD may struggle to obtain childcare and transportation, and psychotherapy may be expensive if not covered by insurance. A potential solution to several of these obstacles is psychotherapy delivered via the Internet. Brief, Internet-delivered, interpersonal psychotherapy showed promising results when used with patients suffering from PPD, particularly in low-income populations [35,37]. Other alternatives to individual psychotherapy include group psychotherapy and mindfulness-based cognitive behavioral therapy, which have shown significant improved mental health outcomes [38].

Medications as treatment for postpartum depression

Although psychotherapy and lifestyle changes are the first choices in the treatment of mild PPD, medication should be considered in the initial treatment of moderate to severe PPD. It should be noted that the USPSTF has found insufficient data to recommend or withhold recommendations on the use of antidepressant medication, on the basis that benefits, and harms, were not well studied [5]. The risk/benefit ratio for both the patient with PPD and the newborn must be evaluated, particularly as many medications are found in human breastmilk.

Providers have used combinations of antidepressant medications, psychotherapy, and other modalities to treat MDDs, including PPD. Treatments have included ECT and hormonal treatments, and repeated transcranial magnetic stimulation (rTMS) as adjuncts to treatment [39,40].

Medications in common use for the treatment of PPD include selective serotonin reuptake inhibitors (SSRIs), serotonin and norepinephrine reuptake inhibitors, and hormone metabolite analogues (Table 2). Tricyclic antidepressants, although still listed as treatments for PPD, are in less common use related to the limited information on the effects on the newborn.

Although there is limited understanding of the underlying causes of PPD, hormonal changes have been a focus of causative theories. In 2019, Zulresso (Brexanolone), an exogenous analogue of a major metabolite of progesterone, was approved for the treatment of moderate to severe PPD [39]. An important

Table 2
Medications used to treat postpartum depression

Medication classification	Example	Comments
Selective serotonin reuptake inhibitors* (SSRIs) *Note: Paroxetine is not used because of potential side effects on the fetus or newborn [4].	Citalopram (Celexa) Fluoxetine (Prozac)	Excreted in human breastmilk, breastfeeding not recommended, or if used, use caution
Selective norepinephrine reuptake inhibitors (SNRIs)	Bupropion (Wellbutrin) Venlafaxine (Effexor)	Excreted in human breast milk. Potential for serious adverse reaction in infants. Breastfeeding contraindicated
Hormone metabolite analogue	Zulresso (Brexanolone)	Food and Drug Administration approved. Given intravenously, requires hospitalization, careful clinical oversight required

Data from Limandri BJ. Postpartum Depression: When the Stakes Are the Highest. J Psychosoc Nurs Ment Health Serv 2019; 57(11): 9-14.

limitation is that Brexanolone, given via a 60-h continuous intravenous infusion, requires inpatient care and can result in dizziness and sudden loss of consciousness [39].

Transcranial magnetic stimulation

A recent addition to the range of treatments for depression is rTMS, approved for treatment for use with MDD. The treatments involve directing an electromagnetic pulse to a specific brain region daily over the course of multiple weeks. Anesthesia is not necessary; there is no pain involved, and the patient remains awake during treatments. These treatments pose no exposure risk to breastfeeding infants. Application of rTMS to treat PPD appears to show sustained improvement in mood at 3 and 6 months after treatment [41]. Previous work has shown that a combination of SSRI and rTMS can be effective in treating PPD [42]. However, drawbacks include the need for limited availability and limited insurance coverage for this new therapy.

Electroconvulsive therapy

ECT is known to be effective for treating MDD. However, it is associated with several adverse effects, including headaches, memory deficits, and recovery from general anesthesia, with each treatment. Therefore, ECT is a less desirable treatment choice for PPD [41]. Although women treated with ECT had a somewhat lower risk of relapse, the negative image of ECT from films and reports can prevent appropriate patients with PPD from agreeing to this treatment. It can be difficult for appropriate patients to agree to this treatment. Insurance coverage, babysitting needs, and transportation issues also can play a part in dissuading likely candidates to this treatment.

Homeopathy

Homeopathy is a therapeutic system based on the theory that a disease can be successfully treated by administering a substance that produces similar symptoms in healthy people. However, despite some interest, there is little information on this method in the treatment of PPD [42].

Supplements and hormones

Considering that the exact biological cause of PPD is yet unknown, identifying supplements or hormones that will decrease this disorder may be unfounded. However, many studies have focused on these areas of research. There has been some research on treating PPD with replacement hormones (progesterone and allopregnanolone), thyroxine, and dietary supplements, including docosahexaenoic acid, essential fatty acids, selenium, calcium, zinc, magnesium, vitamin D and tryptophan, tyrosine, and blueberry [27]. However, the research on this area is preliminary, and recommendations are elusive.

POSTPARTUM PSYCHOSIS TREATMENT

PPP is the least common, yet the most devastating of all the subcategories of perinatal affective disorders. It occurs in less than 3 per 1000 women and is characterized by an abrupt onset of severe symptoms that may begin immediately after delivery until 4 weeks postpartum, and that deteriorate rapidly, including hallucinations, delusions, and suicidal and infanticidal urges [43]. The severity and rapid onset of symptoms of PPP require all practitioners to understand the potential for danger to the mother and infant, and to be prepared to act immediately should symptoms arise. No patient with PPP should be left alone with an infant or child from the onset of symptoms. Immediate assessment and transfer to inpatient psychiatric services are indicated, where antipsychotic medication is the treatment of choice. Family members will need support during this challenging time and should be involved as the patient improves with medication in care and discharge planning.

DISCUSSION

PPD and related disorders are conditions that all providers should be aware of and assessing for in all pregnant and parenting patients for a full year following birth. Patients whose screens indicate that they are at risk should be referred for group or individual psychotherapy, whether in person or via telehealth. Patients and their family members should receive clear, matter-of-fact information on PPD and be encouraged to contact their provider should symptoms worsen.

Family members or friends should be coached to encourage supportive care of the birth parent to prevent or ameliorate the effects of PPD. Supportive care may include helping with childcare, helping with household tasks, and allowing the patient to talk and have weekly free time away from the baby. The patient's informal support network also may help provide good nutrition and rest time and may encourage regular, moderate exercise after the first few days or weeks postpartum.

Patients should be coached toward realistic expectations of early postpartum and newborn care and should be encouraged to think through resources they may have for help before such resources are needed. Parenting groups for parents of infants, online or in person, may be used for some support.

Patients who have moderate to severe or worsening symptoms of PPD should be started on an approved antidepressant after considering risks and benefits to the patient and the baby and referred to psychiatric care. Any patients with PPP should be referred for acute care at once, and the baby or other children kept in a safe, supervised situation.

SUMMARY

PPD, a subset of peripartal depression, is a major mental health disorder that affects a significant proportion of postpartum patients. Screening for PPD is an important part of antepartum and postpartum care, and through the first year following delivery. Good informal support from family, friends, or social groups may prevent some PPD and may ameliorate the effects on the family constellation. However, patients whose screens may indicate PPD should be referred promptly for psychotherapy and medication, and other adjunct therapies should be considered.

CLINICS CARE POINTS

- PPD impacts the entire family constellation, particularly the birthing parent and the newborn. Support and monitoring of all family members including the infant is essential.
- Symptoms of PPD may look like other types of depression and may include anxiety symptoms. Additional symptoms may include sleeplessness, lack of appetite, and panic in addition to typical depressive symptoms.
- PPD may occur longer than the initial 6 weeks postpartum. Affective disorders can manifest during pregnancy and through the first year of newborn life.
- Symptoms of psychosis in the postpartum patient is a crisis situation. Patients require emergency evaluation, and newborns and children must not be left alone with patients under any circumstances.

Disclosure

K. Green has no disclosures of any commercial or financial conflicts of interest and no funding sources related to this work. M. Low has no disclosures of any commercial or financial conflicts of interest and no funding sources related to this work.

References

1 Segre L, Davis W. Postpartum depression and perinatal mood disorders in the DSM. In Mayo Clinic.. Available at: https://www.postpartum.net/wp-content/uploads/2014/11/DSM-5-Summary-PSI.pdf. Accessed August 15, 2021.

2 American Psychiatric Association. Diagnostic and statistical manual of mental disorders (DSM-5). 5th edition. Washington (DC): American Psychiatric Association; 2013.

3 Major depressive disorder with peripartum onset. In: National Alliance on Mental Illness (NAMI). Available at: https://www.nami.org/About-Mental-Illness/Mental-Health-Conditions/Depression/Major-Depressive-Disorder-with-Peripartum-Onset. Accessed August 21, 2021.

4 Torres F. What is postpartum depression? Depression during pregnancy and after childbirth. In: American Psychiatric Association. Available at: https://www.psychiatry.org/patients-families/postpartum-depression/what-is-postpartum-depression. Accessed August 17, 2021.

5 Perinatal depression: preventive interventions. In: U.S. Preventative Task Force Services. Available at: https://www.uspreventiveservicestaskforce.org/uspstf/recommendation/perinatal-depression-preventive-interventions#bootstrap-panel–4. Accessed August 17, 2021.

6 Trends in pregnancy and childbirth complications in the U.S. In: Blue Cross Blue Shield Association. Available at: https://www.bcbs.com/the-health-of-america/reports/trends-in-pregnancy-and-childbirth-complications-in-the-us. Accessed August 18, 2021.

7 Shorey S, Chee CYI, Ng ED, et al. Prevalence and incidence of postpartum depression among healthy mothers: a systematic review and meta-analysis. J Psychiatr Res 2018;104: 235–48.

8 Loudon I. Puerperal insanity in the 19th century. J R Soc Med 1988;81(2):76–9.

9 Buist A. Childhood abuse, postpartum depression and parenting difficulties: a literature review of associations. Aust N Z J Psychiatry 1998;32(3):370–8.

10 Beck CT. A checklist to identify women at risk for developing postpartum depression. J Obstet Gynecol Neonatal Nurs 1998;27(1):39–46.

11 Postpartum depression. In: OASH Office on Women's Health website, Health and Human Services. 2019. Available at: https://www.womenshealth.gov/mental-health/mental-health-conditions/postpartum-depression. Accessed August 27, 2021.

12 Heron J, McGuinness M, Blackmore ER, et al. Early postpartum symptoms in puerperal psychosis. BJOG 2008;115:348–53.

13 Sorg M, Coddington J, Ahmed A, et al. Improving postpartum depression screening in pediatric primary care: a quality improvement project. J Pediatr Nurs 2019;46:83–8.

14 Sit D, Rothschild AJ, Wisner KL. A review of postpartum psychosis. J Womens Health 2006;15:352–68.

15 Kirchengast S. The insane woman-mental disorders and female life history-a Darwinian approach. Neuropsychiatry 2016;6:286–97.

16 Tichenor V, McQuillan J, Greil AL, et al. Variation in attitudes toward being a mother by race/ethnicity and education among women in the United States. Sociol Perspect 2017;60(3):600–19.

17 Liu CH, Giallo R, Doan SN, et al. Racial and ethnic differences in prenatal life stress and postpartum depression symptoms. Arch Psychiatr Nurs 2016;30(1):7–12.

18 Sakowicz A, Matovina CN, Imeroni SK, et al. The association between the COVID-19 pandemic and postpartum care provision. AJOG MFM 2021;3(6):100460.

19 Panchal N, Kamal R, Cox C, et al. The implications of COVID-19 for mental health and substance use. In KFF. Available at: https://www.kff.org/coronavirus-covid-19/issue-brief/the-implications-of-covid-19-for-mental-health-and-substance-use/. Accessed August 20, 2021.

20 Keys to the diagnosis of postpartum depression. In Mayo Clinic Proc. Available at: https://www.mayoclinicproceedings.org/action/showFullTableHTML?isHtml=true&tableId=tbl1&pii=S0025-6196%2814%2900164-5. Accessed August 27, 2021.

21 Bina R, Harrington D. Differential predictors of postpartum depression and anxiety: the Edinburgh Postnatal Depression Scale Hebrew version two factor structure construct validity. Matern Child Health J 2017;21(12):2237–44.

22 Newland R, Parade S. The Brown Univ Child Adolesc Behav Lett 2016; 32: 1 1058-1073.

23 ACOG Committee Opinion no. 757. Screening for perinatal depression. Obstet Gynecol 2018;132(5):e208–12.

24 Martin CJH, Norris G, Martin CR. Midwives' role in screening for antenatal depression and postnatal depression. Br J Midwifery 2020;28(9):666–72.

25 Forsyth J, Boath E, Henshaw C, et al. Exercise as an adjunct treatment for postpartum depression for women living in an inner city-a pilot study. Health Care Women Int 2017;38(6):635–9.

26 Carter T, Bastounis A, Guo B, et al. The effectiveness of exercise-based interventions for preventing or treating postpartum depression: a systematic review and meta-analysis. Arch Womens Ment Health 2019;22(1):37–53.

27 Dowlati Y, Meyer J. Promising leads and pitfalls: a review of dietary supplements and hormone treatments to prevent postpartum blues and postpartum depression. Arch Womens Ment Health 2021;24:381–9.

28 Pao C, Guintivano J, Santos H, et al. Postpartum depression and social support in a racially and ethnically diverse population of women. Arch Womens Ment Health 2019;22(1):105–14.

29 Woolhouse H, Miller K, Brown SJ, et al. Frequency of "time for self" is a significant predictor of postnatal depressive symptoms: results from a prospective pregnancy cohort study. Birth 2016;43(1):58–67.

30 Fonseca A, Monteiro F, Alves S, et al. Be a mom, a web-based intervention to prevent postpartum depression: results from a pilot randomized controlled trial. Behav Ther 2019;51(4):616–33.

31 Roman M, Constantin T, Bostan CM. The efficiency of online cognitive-behavioral therapy for postpartum depressive symptomatology: a systematic review and meta-analysis. Women Health 2020;60(1):99–112.

32 Ando H, Shen J, Morishige K, et al. Association between postpartum depression and social support satisfaction levels at four months after childbirth. Arch Psychiatr Nurs 2021;35(4): 341–6.

33 ACOG Committee Opinion No. 736: optimizing postpartum care. Obstet Gynecol 2018;131(5):e140–50.

34 Morehead AN. Current recommendations for screening and management of postpartum depression. Women's Healthc A Clin J NPs 2020;8(4):1–9.

35 Loughnan SA, Sie A, Hobbs MJ, et al. A randomized controlled trial of 'MUMentum Pregnancy': internet-delivered cognitive behavioral therapy program for antenatal anxiety and depression. J Affect Disord 2019;243:381–90.

36 Stamou G, García-Palacios A, Botella C. Cognitive-behavioural therapy and interpersonal psychotherapy for the treatment of post-natal depression: a narrative review. BMC Psychol 2018;6.

37 Lenze S, Potts M. Brief interpersonal psychotherapy for depression during pregnancy in a low-income population: a randomized controlled trial. J Affect Disord 2017;210:151–7.

38 Shulman B, Dueck R, Ryan D, et al. Feasibility of a mindfulness-based cognitive therapy group intervention as an adjunctive treatment for postpartum depression and anxiety. J Affect Disord 2018;235:61–7.

39 Powell JG, Garland S, Preston K, et al. Brexanolone (Zulresso): finally, an FDA-approved treatment for postpartum depression. Ann Pharmacother 2020;54(2):157–63.

40 Limandri BJ. Postpartum depression: when the stakes are the highest. J Psychosoc Nurs Ment Health Serv 2019;57(11):9–14.

41 Cox EQ, Killenberg S, Frische R, et al. Repetitive transcranial magnetic stimulation for the treatment of postpartum depression. J Affect Disord 2020;264(1):193–200.

42 Zhang Y, Zhang T, Tong CY, et al. Effect of repeated transcranial magnetic stimulation combined with antidepressant drugs on cognitive function and breastfeeding of postpartum depression patients. Int J Psychiatry 2018;45:323–6.

43 Forde R, Peters S, Wittkowski A. Recovery from postpartum psychosis: a systematic review and meta synthesis of women's and families' experiences. Arch Womens Ment Health 2020;23(5):597–612.

Measuring the Impact of Health Literacy on Perinatal Depression

Nicole Lynne Audritsh, DNP, CNM

Wayne State University, 5557 Cass Avenue, #142, Detroit, MI 48202, USA

Keywords

• Health literacy • Perinatal depression • Postpartum depression • Literacy
• Medical mistrust • Gender bias

Key points

• Depression is the third leading cause of disease burden in the world for women, and individuals with low health literacy are 2 times more likely to experience depression symptoms than individuals with adequate health literacy skills.

• A pregnant person's ability to find and understand information related to their pregnancy, their physical and emotional health, and the health of their baby is critical to the decision-making process.

• Evaluation of a person's health literacy is important during pregnancy because this represents a time when people are exposed to excessive amounts of health information and possibly motivated to make significant health behavior changes.

• As clinicians caring for patients at risk for perinatal depression, we can advocate for and promote health literacy for individual mental health improvement as well as contribute to overall improvement in decreasing maternal mortality in the United States by assessing for health literacy and working to intervene where appropriate.

INTRODUCTION

Depression is the third leading cause of disease burden in the world for women [1], and individuals with low health literacy are 2 times more likely to experience depression symptoms than individuals with adequate health literacy skills [2]. Research suggests that people who feel empowered in their decisions during pregnancy have higher health literacy and a much lower risk of perinatal depression than their counterparts [3,4]. The perinatal period, pregnancy through 1-year after childbirth, can be a particularly vulnerable time when

E-mail address: Bv8083@wayne.edu

https://doi.org/10.1016/j.yfpn.2021.12.010
2589-420X/22/© 2021 Elsevier Inc. All rights reserved.

people often experience major physical, emotional, hormonal, and social changes [3]. Perinatal depression is common during the 12 months following birth, affecting 10% to 15% of those who experience pregnancy and childbirth [3].

Patients who are pregnant or postpartum are vulnerable for major and minor depressive episodes [3]. Major or minor depression during pregnancy, or during the postpartum period of the first 12 months following delivery, is diagnosed as perinatal depression. Depressive episodes during this time can have devastating consequences not only for the person experiencing this but also for the infant and the family, including both mother and father [3]. It can lead to compromised bonding for the mother and infant, ineffective integration of the infant into the family as well as maternal and paternal anxiety and depression [3].

PREVALENCE

The prevalence of perinatal depression is a significant cost to individuals, children, families, and the communities. In 2011, 10% of postpartum women met criteria for perinatal depression and major depressive disorders, making it even more important that clinicians perform screenings within the first year postpartum for depression [5]. Women in the perinatal period will be seen in nurse practitioner clinics for any number of reasons, including primary care, acute care visits, health promotion reasons, family planning visits, and postpartum care. In the United States in 2013, there was $2.4 trillion spent on health care treatments including individuals out of pocket costs for mental health care [6]. Mental health and substance abuse disorders rank number 4 in the cost category, with $187.8 billion dollars spent in 2013, ranking behind cardiovascular diseases; diabetes, urogenital, blood, and endocrine diseases; and neurologic diseases including Alzheimer disease [6]. Depressive disorders are listed as the sixth most costly health condition behind diabetes mellitus, ischemic heart disease, low back and neck pain, hypertension, and injuries due to falls [6].

PERINATAL DEPRESSION

Symptoms of perinatal depression include, but are not limited to, feelings of hopelessness, pessimism, worthlessness, difficulty concentrating, as well as suicidal ideation, thoughts, and attempts [3]. If left untreated, perinatal depression not only affects their health but also adversely affect the infant's mental health and development [3]. A pregnant person's ability to find and understand information related to their pregnancy, their physical and emotional health, and the health of their baby is critical to the decision-making process [7].

Women are twice as likely to suffer from mood and anxiety disorders in their lifetimes when compared with men, and their risk for mood disorders increases during the perinatal period [8]. In addition, young, low-income women, with low literacy rates, living in urban areas are disproportionally affected by depression during the perinatal time period when compared with women who do not live in urban areas [9]. Perinatal depression is associated with poor maternal well-being, neonatal outcomes, disruptions in maternal-fetal attachment, interruptions in breastfeeding initiation, and impairments in fetal development [1,8]. Because this is a time of maternal-infant attachment and a transition to motherhood, perinatal depression can and often does affect women with lifelong symptoms such as depression and anxiety as well as interrupted maternal infant bonding [3].

Perinatal depression is listed as one of the key indicators in the fight against maternal mortality. Maternal mortality is currently one of the World Health Organization's (WHO's) key agenda items and lists the rate as highly unacceptable [10]. Approximately 295,000 women died during and following childbirth in the year 2017, and most of these deaths occurred in settings that could have been prevented. The settings in which nurse practitioners see women and could have impacts on the maternal mortality rate are during office visits in the following time frames: antepartum, well woman care, postpartum, and during health promotion visits. The WHO lists the following factors that prevent women from receiving or seeking care during pregnancy and childbirth: poverty, distance to facilities, inadequate and cultural beliefs and services, and finally lack of information, perhaps due to a lack of understanding due to health literacy [10]. In addition, research suggests that health literacy barriers, such as poor knowledge about treatment options and symptoms of depression, have been identified as one of the most important obstacles to seeking professional help during the perinatal period [8].

HEALTH LITERACY DURING PREGNANCY

Health literacy is the degree to which an individual can obtain, process, and understand the basic health information and services they need to make informed and appropriate health-related decisions; this includes the ability to read, write, interpret, and understand information that is talked about and given to them in clinic with their clinician [11]. In addition, it includes information that women read on the Internet, hear from friends and family members, and read in books about pregnancy, childbirth, and motherhood [12]. Health literacy describes the level of knowledge, personal skills, and confidence of a woman to take action in their life to improve personal and community health by changing their lifestyle and living conditions [1].

Health literacy is also identified as accurate health information and services that people can easily find, understand, and use to inform their decisions and action. Because health literacy is such an important piece of a patients' well-being, the American College of Obstetrics and Gynecology released a Committee Opinion highlighting the need for consideration of patients' health literacy skills for health promotion and clinical care activities [13]. In addition, women are exposed to significant health information, health care providers, and online and written educational materials, making this an optimal time to assess and evaluate a woman's health literacy [14].

HEALTH LITERACY AND PERINATAL DEPRESSION

Women with low health literacy are more likely to experience increased high rates of birth trauma, unpleasant birth experiences, less understanding of conditions and complications during pregnancy, and increased mental health diagnoses [7,13,15]. Women with low health literacy are also more likely to have issues completing activities of daily living, limitations in activities of daily living, as well as a lower mental health status altogether [16]. Although health literacy is recognized as a more reliable predictor of maternal health and birth outcomes than socioeconomic status or race [14,17], little is known about the link between health literacy and perinatal depression, except that women with low health literacy are at much higher risk of experiencing perinatal depression than women with higher literacy levels. Evaluation of a person's health literacy is important during pregnancy because this represents a time when people are exposed to excessive amounts of health information and possibly motivated to make significant health behavior changes [14]. During this time of sensitive decision-making and health information intake, clinicians can thread health literacy into their care planning throughout every step. Studies suggest integrating health literacy promotion via mobile application, on-demand patient education, and individual counseling provided by health care professionals are suggested best practices for promotion of health literacy during pregnancy [7].

Without adequate health literacy, it is possible that women lack the ability to recognize symptoms of perinatal depression and seek treatment when necessary. Research suggests that people with higher rates of health literacy would have lower impacts of perinatal depression as they would recognize symptoms sooner and seek treatment in a shorter time frame [8]. The purpose of this literature review is to explore the literature surrounding health literacy and perinatal depression.

METHODS

A comprehensive literature search was performed using the keywords of postpartum depression/perinatal depression AND health literacy. Four databases were used: MEDLINE, CINAHL, Scopus, and PubMed. Inclusion criteria were: (a) original research, (b) pregnant or had a baby within the last 12 months, and (c) sample consists of adult women over 16 years of age. Exclusion criteria were: (a) antenatal depression and major depression-focused research studies, and (b) books. The search in each database was limited to English language, peer-reviewed publications, academic journals, and published between 2015 and 2020.

The computer search, based on English language, peer reviewed, and academic journals, initially yielded 47 articles, of which 20 were duplicates. After reviewing the titles and abstracts of the remaining 27 articles based on inclusion and exclusion criteria, the number of articles was decreased to 16 articles. After reviewing the full article, 7 articles were found to focus on health literacy and perinatal depression (Table 1).

Table 1
Literature review results

Reference	Data Collection/Time Points	Sample/Setting	Instruments	Results
Amipara et al., [18] 2020	Postpartum women	Cross-sectional study among 116 postpartum women between ages 20 and30 y attending the Anganwadi centers under the Urban Health Training Centre area of Medical College of Valsad district. A purposive sampling was applied.	• Edinburgh postpartum depression scale (EPDS) • WHO Infant and Young Child Feeding guidelines • WHO growth charts	Found a statistically significant (P<.05) association between health literacy and perinatal depression. Based on the findings of this study, it was recommended that early prevention and intervention be instituted so that referral and treatment can be initiated before harm is reached at the level of the mother or the child.
Fonseca et al, [8] 2017	32.5% pregnant 67.5% postnatally	194 women 82% married/cohabitating 71%/8% employed	• EPDS • Depression literacy questionnaire (D-Lit) • Difficulties in emotional regulation (DERS) • Awareness/recognition of psychopathological symptoms	66 women (34%) presented with clinically significant psychopathological symptoms, with 65.15% presenting with EPDS scores of >12. 59.1% of women (n = 39) were aware of their symptoms. Lower education levels are associated with poor *(continued on next page)*

Table 1
(continued)

Reference	Data Collection/Time Points	Sample/Setting	Instruments	Results
				depression literacy in women during the perinatal depression period.
Mirsalimi et al, [20] 2020	Study 1: perinatal Study 2: perinatal	Study 1: 15 women Study 2: 692 women	• Postpartum depression literacy scale (PoDLiS)	Findings showed that overall women did not have adequate knowledge about postpartum depression and most respondents said they would get their information about perinatal depression from the Internet.
Poreddi et al, [27,28] 2020	Hindu family members from a government run hospital in Bangalore, South India. Ages 18–65 y.	n = 202 family members	Qualitative study	Adequate knowledge among family members was instrumental in the mother receiving the help she needed when she has perinatal depression symptoms. Participants with less education had negative attitudes including feeling shame that the woman had postpartum depression than

Recto & Champion, [21] 2017	Hispanic female adolescents	Between the ages of 15 and 19 y	Convenience sample cross-sectional design	participants who had more education. Suggest the need to improve health literacy. Adolescents reported perinatal depressions had high health literacy scores, indicating greater ability to recognize mental health disorders. Those who report perinatal depression had significantly higher mental health literacy than those without perinatal depression. This article also reinforces the distrust between patients and providers and the need for intense trust and relationship building with the provider and patient to provide the most competent care.
Recto [22], 2019	Pregnant and postpartum women	20 Between the ages of 15 and 19 y	Qualitative study	Revealed that the women in this community relied on what other women thought about perinatal depression when considering asking for help. If other women felt (continued on next page)

Table 1
(continued)

Reference	Data Collection/Time Points	Sample/Setting	Instruments	Results
				that the perinatal depression was not happening, then the original woman was reluctant to ask for help. Women are getting the information about perinatal depression from other women, not from their providers because of a lack of trust.
Swami et al, [19] 2020	Adult patients	406 adults Ages 18–70 y; 92% white	Qualitative study	Findings suggested that participants were significantly more likely to indicate something was wrong when the target was female, rather than male indicating there may be a gender bias. In addition, there was very poor recognition of paternal perinatal depression, and more education about this in the public may benefit the health literacy of men in our communities.

| Wagner et al, [29] 2020 | Low-income Hispanic, White, and African American postpartum women from 2 health care settings | 21 adult women | Qualitative study | Most women reported seeking additional information during their pregnancy about postpartum care from the Internet. In addition, they reported comparing advice they received from their doctor with Internet advice. Just more than half the women stated that they did not have time to read the information that was sent home with them and spent that time focusing on the baby and themselves. The main take away from this study was that 43% of the participants indicated a need for postpartum depression education and stated that it was the topic that received the least referral and advice on potential treatment and resources at discharge from the hospital. |

RESULTS

Seven studies were identified that presented quantitative and qualitative findings on the impact of health literacy on patients with postpartum depression. Two of them produced statistically significant findings that linked lower education levels to health literacy and postpartum depression. Three of them discussed the lack of knowledge and mental health literacy women had about postpartum depression and where their information was obtained. One discussed gender bias and the impact of perinatal depression on paternal figures.

LOWER EDUCATION LEVELS ASSOCIATED WITH POOR DEPRESSION LITERACY

According to Fonseca, there is a direct correlation between the education level of a woman and the ability to recognize depression signs and symptoms [8]. In the 2017 study, Edinburgh Depression Scale questionnaires were given along with Depression Literacy Scales and Difficulties in Emotional Regulation Scales, and an awareness/recognition of psychopathological symptoms question was asked. The total number of participants in this study was 194, and 66 of them presented clinically significant for being aware of their psychopathological symptoms. Women's depression literacy concerning treatment was significantly correlated with education ($P = .40$), income ($P = .26$), psychiatric treatment ($P = .18$), and psychiatric history ($P = .24$) [8]. Specifically, this means that when a woman is poorer, less educated, and has a lower household income with no prior psychiatric history or treatment, she will have a lower level of depression literacy.

In a 2020 cross-sectional study in which the research was focused on 116 postpartum mothers irrespective of their socioeconomic status where the team used the Edinburgh Postpartum Scale (EPDS), The WHO Infant and Young Child Feeding Guidelines and the WHO growth charts to assess nutritional status for infants [18]. Along with this research, however, they asked about health literacy. There was a statistical significance ($p \leq 0.05$) of women who were not literate in this study in which 7% of the women were found to be depressed per the EPDS [18].

Lower literacy levels can lead to higher rates of untreated perinatal depression rates, as the patients are unable to recognize their symptoms and their need for treatment. In addition, these patients are often the ones with the least amount of social support and therefore at additional high risk for perinatal depression.

GENDER BIAS

According to a 2020 qualitative study, there is evidence that there may be a gender bias at work to mental health literacy [19]. This qualitative study consisted of 406 British men and women ranging in age from 18 to 70 years. The individuals were presented with case vignettes and were then asked if "anything was wrong" with the individuals described. The respondents were then asked in an open-ended question what they believed was wrong. They were also asked to judge on a 7-point scale how distressing they believed the condition were and how likely they would be to suggest that the targets seek help for their problems [19].

The results were very interesting. Women and men were likely to indicate that something was wrong with the female target and the most common description was postnatal/postpartum depression (92.9%) and baby blues (5.6%). Of those who believed that there was something wrong with the male target, the most common response was perinatal depression (61.2%). Overall, 90.1% of the participants correctly identify the female population as having perinatal depression, yet with the male population, only 46.3% of the participants are described as having perinatal depression [19]. There is obviously a gender bias happening here, perhaps a stereotype that perinatal depression only or disproportionately affects women due to gender-specific factors, birth factors, hormonal reasons, breastfeeding, and pregnancy-related symptoms [19]. It is also possible that attention to male perinatal depression receives very little support and awareness and therefore is not well thought of; therefore, men are perceived as less likely to experience symptoms of mental health disorders.

Much more work should be done to promote awareness toward the adjustment to parenthood that men experience and the possibility of perinatal mood disorders that men are at risk for. Men should be assessed for health literacy as well as perinatal depression. The adjustment period after having a newborn baby is an adjustment for everyone who is living with that child and can be overwhelming and the man may not feel confident in asking for help, and this may be missed by health care providers in routine assessments of new parents [19]. In addition to feeling overwhelmed, having a lack of health literacy can cause the man to not recognize his symptoms right away, therefore leading him not to seek help in a timely manner.

MEDICAL MISTRUST IN THE MEDICAL COMMUNITY

Possibly the most important theme to come out of this literature review is the lack of medical trust and the impact on perinatal mood disorders. The literature suggests that women are retrieving information on the Internet and obtaining information from family and friends, rather than seeking information from their physicians because of medical mistrust [20–26]. It is imperative that the medical community addresses this medical mistrust and works to counteract it to improve the perinatal depression and health literacy outcomes improve.

According to Mirsalimi and colleagues [20], most women are obtaining their information about depression from the Internet, and most women are not proactively seeking treatment during the postpartum period. The lack of knowledge about perinatal depression symptoms and treatment options are a major help-seeking barrier indicating how significant the health literacy role is in the treatment process. An early intervention that clinicians can implement to counteract medical mistrust is early depression screening. Having conversations early and often about depression facilitates open and honest conversations with patients that allow for relationships full of trust [20]. Some patients are afraid to disclose depression to health care providers because of the fear that their information will be shared, so ensuring that the clinic spaces are private, quiet, and safe is another intervention that clinicians can do in order to create trustful relationships for patients [20]. Finally, research tells us that patients need to feel connected to clinicians to reveal their depression, so ensuring relationship-based care is of utmost importance to establishing a rapport with them [20].

Ensuring that a patient has trust in their provider is critically important to their health and their health literacy. If the patient does not trust their provider, they will not tell them information and they will not listen to or invest in resources that are given to them by that provider. It is critical that the provider and the office staff invest in the patient and gaining their trust to become a safe medical home for them. Allowing adequate time for appointments, sitting down on the patients' level during visits and looking the patient in the eyes while speaking with them, performing the EPDS and reviewing it with the patient while asking open-ended questions and being an open safe space for patients to reveal their feelings and thoughts without rushing through appointments are some suggestions for creating trusting relationships with patients.

In addition, assessing for health literacy is a good way to ensure open communication is occurring between the patient and the provider. By administering the Test of Functional Health Literacy Tool (TOFHLA) in clinic, an office can ensure that the patients' needs are being met, as far as communications needs go. This assessment should occur during the initial intake of a patient or whenever this procedure is started in the office. It is a 36-item questionnaire and is a measure of the patients' ability to read and understand health care information. It should be given in an area that will allow for complete privacy and 15 minutes of quiet time. There are directions for administration and scoring included with the examination. Our ability to communicate follow-up care to a patient completely depends on the patients' ability to read and comprehend the directions that we dispense to them. It is imperative that we start this process by understanding where the patient is in literacy level.

SUMMARY

Assessment of literacy levels during initial intake of patients in clinics is part of identifying patient needs and improving patient outcomes. Once a clinician is aware of a patients' literacy level, they can then plan for their care in a more comprehensive and dutiful way. Measuring health literacy along with measuring perinatal depression with the EDPS is imperative. There is an International Classification of Diseases-10 code for low level of literacy that can be billed along with the visit: Z55.0 Low level of Literacy. American College of Obstetrics and Gynecologists recommends that women in the postpartum state should be screened for postpartum depression at 6 weeks using the EPDS at any time that the patient is seen for any reason in our care. Although we are assessing for postpartum depression, clinicians need to remember that this is a good time to assess for health literacy, especially knowing that there is so much information being given to the patient at this point, she is vulnerable, and her outcomes depend on her ability to comprehend what we are telling her.

Health literacy is critical for maternal and infant outcomes in the maternal health field. It can hinder women's access, understanding, and ability to make informed decisions during pregnancy, ultimately affecting their maternal and neonatal outcomes. Especially when considering that health literacy is recognized a key determinant of health and an even more reliable predictor of maternal health and birth outcomes than socioeconomic status, age, or race, clinicians need to be focusing on the health literacy of their patients at all points in care.

Advanced practice nurses are in a position of often being the initial access to health care and may see patients in the office or hospital setting admission, through discharge. As clinicians caring for patients at risk for perinatal depression, we can advocate for and promote health literacy for individual mental health improvement as well as contribute to overall improvement in decreasing maternal mortality in the United States by assessing for health literacy and working to intervene where appropriate.

CLINICS CARE POINTS

- APRN's are in a position to advocate for health l iteracy screening in their clinics to promote improved outcomes for maternal and infant mortality.Health literacy is a recognized key determinant of health and a better indicator of maternal health and birth outcomes than socioecnomic status, age, and race.
- Utilizing EDPS and TOFHLA as part of initial patient intake documents in a clinic's paperwork is a step in the right direction to assessing health literacy and ensuring open communication between providers and patients.

References

[1] Madlala SS, Kassier SM. Antenatal and postpartum depression: effects of infant and young child health and feeding practices. South Afr J Clin Nutr 2018;31(1):1–7.

[2] Cramer RJ, Long MM, Jenkins J, et al. A systematic review of intervnetions for healthcare professionals to improve screening and referral for perinatal mood and anxiety disorders. Arch Womens Ment Health 2019;22(1):25–36.

[3] American Psychological Association. Postpartum depression 2008. Available at: https://www.apa.org/pi/women/resources/reports/postpartum-depression August 1, 2021.

[4] Morgenlander MA, Tyrrell H, Garfunkel LC, et al. Screening for social determinants of health in pediatric resident continuity clinic. Acad Pediatr 2019;19(8):868–74.

[5] American College of Obstetricians and Gynecologists. Screening for perinatal depression. 2018. Available at: http://acog.org/clinical/clinical-guidance/committee-opinion/articles/2018/11/screening-for-perinatal-depression?utm_source=redirect&utm_medium=web&utm_campaign=otn#:~:text=Theprevalenceofperinataldepressionisasignificant,metthecriteri August 18, 2021.

[6] American Psychological Association. By the numbers: The cost of treatment. 2021. Available at: https://www.apa.org/monitor/2017/03/numbers August 18, 2021.

[7] Hussey L, Frazer C, Kopulos MI. Impact of health literacy in educating pregnant millennial women. Int J Childbirth Education 2019;31(3):13–8.

[8] Fonseca A, Silva S, Canavarro MC. Depression Literacy and Awareness of Psychopathological symptoms during the perinatal period. J Obstet Gynecol Neonatal Nurses 2017;46(2): 197–208.

[9] Chaudron LH. Accuracy of depression screening tools for identifying postpartum depression among urban mothers. Pediatrics 2010;125:609–17.

[10] World health organization. Maternal mortality 2020. Available at: https://www.who.int/news-room/fact-sheets/detail/maternal-mortality April 8, 2021.

[11] CDC. Healthy People 2030. National Center for Health Statistics. 2020. Available at: https://www.cdc.gov/nchs/healthy_people/index.htm April 8, 2021.

[12] Muhange MJ, Mulango JR. The what, why and how of health literacy: A systematic review of literature. Int J Health 2017;5(2):107–14.

[13] Kilfoyle KA, Vitko M, O'Conor R, et al. Health literacy and women's reproductive health: A systematic review. J Womens Health 2016;25:12.

[14] Vamos CA, Thompson EL, Griner SB, et al. Applying organizational health literacy to maternal and child health. Matern Child Health J 2019;23(5):597–602.

[15] Senol DK, Goi I, Ozkan SA. The effect of health literacy levels of pregnant women receiving prenatal care: A cross sectional descriptive study. Int J Caring Sci 2019;2(3):1717–24.

[16] Wolf MS, Gazmararian JA, Baker DW. Health literacy and functional health status in Korean older adults. J Clin Nurs 2009;18(16):2337–43. Available at:.

[17] Speros C. Health Literacy: A Concept Analysis. J Adv Nurs 2005;50(6):633–40.

[18] Amipara T, Baria H, Nayak S. A study on postpartum depression and its association with infant feeding practices and infant nutritional status among mothers attending the anganwadi centers of valsad district, gujarat, india. Indian J Community Med 2020;45(3): 299–302.

[19] Swami V, Barron D, Smith L, et al. Mental health literacy of maternal and paternal postnatal (postpartum) depression in british adults. J Ment Health 2020;29(2):217–24.

[20] Mirsalimi F, Ghofranipour F, Noroozi A, et al. The postpartum depression literacy scale (PoDLiS): Development and psychometric properties. BMC Pregnancy Childbirth 2020;20(1):1–13.

[21] Recto P, Champion JD. Assessment of mental health literacy among perinatal hispanic adolescents. Issues Ment Health Nurs 2017;38(12):1030–8.

[22] Recto P. Mexican-American adolescents' views on factors that facilitate recognition and help-seeking for perinatal depression. Issues Ment Health Nurs 2019;40(9):821–4.

[23] Gazmararian J, Baker D, Parker R. A multivariate analysis of factors associated with depression: evaluating the role of health literacy as a potential contributor. Arch Intern Med 2000;160:3307–14.

[24] Mancuso J. Health literacy: a concept/dimensional analysis. Nurs Health Sci 2008;10: 248–55.

[25] Moshki M, Baloochi Beydokhti T, Cheravi K. The effect of educational intervention on prevention of postpartum depression: an application of health locus of control. J Clin Nurs 2014;23:15–6.

[26] Organization, W. H. World Health Organization. World Health Organization: Health Promotion. 2020.

[27] Poreddi V, Thomas B, Paulose B, et al. Knowledge and attitudes of family members towards postpartum depression. Arch Psychiatr Nurs 2020; https://doi.org/10.1016/j.apnu.2020.09.003.

[28] Sluijs AM, Cleiren MPHD, van Lith JMM, et al. Is fear of childbirth related to the woman's preferred location for giving birth? A Dutch low-risk cohort study. Birth 2020;47(1): 144–52.

[29] Wagner T, Thompson EL, Gadson A, et al. Postpartum education and health literacy: New moms' perspectives. J Consumer Health Internet 2020;24(4):346–59.

Pediatrics

The Good, the Bad, and the Potential

Best Practices for Navigating Technology Use Among Pediatric Populations

Lisa Militello, PhD, MPH, RN, CPNP[a],*,
Elizabeth Hutson, PhD, APRN-CNP, PMHNP-BC[b]

[a]The Ohio State University, College of Nursing, 1585 Neil Avenue, Columbus, OH 43210, USA;
[b]Texas Tech University Health Sciences Center, School of Nursing, 3601 4th Street, Lubbock, TX 79430, USA

Keywords

• Adolescent • Child • Family • Communication • Bullying • Technology • Apps
• Primary care

Key points

• Children, teens, and families continue to use and adopt various technologies, making this a critically important topic for health supervision.

• Parents and children look to health care providers for reliable technology-based guidance and resources to foster health and well-being.

• Expert guidelines need to be reconciled with real-world technology use, recognizing that technology use among children and parents is interrelated, and there are both benefits and risks to technology use.

• Providers can temper clinical guidelines by focusing on child development and discussing quality of technology use.

• Implicit bias is one area clinicians can improve to support technology use among children and families, recognizing that not all technology is "bad" and that discussions focused on quality over quantity may lead to productive conversations with families.

*Corresponding author. E-mail address: Militello.14@osu.edu

https://doi.org/10.1016/j.yfpn.2021.12.011
2589-420X/22/© 2022 Elsevier Inc. All rights reserved.

INTRODUCTION

Over the past 2 decades there has been a dramatic increase in technology use across diverse populations, including children and teens. Prepandemic, 95% of teens (ages 13–17 years) reported having a smartphone and 45% reported being online "almost constantly" [1]. Teens and tweens most often used social media, specifically YouTube (85%), Instagram (72%), and Snapchat (35%). Nearly 72% of all Americans have reported using some form of social media [2]. Similarly, among children younger than 8 years, nearly half (48%) of children reported having their own mobile device (eg, tablet, smartphone), most commonly a tablet (61%). Video viewing (both educational and recreational) and gaming accounted for most of the screen time use in children younger than 8 years. Children ages 2 to 4 years averaged 2.5 h/d in front of screens and children ages 5 to 8 years averaged 3 h/d, consisting mostly of viewing videos, reading/doing homework, or video chatting [3].

Differences in technology use by race/ethnicity and income were also prominent before the pandemic. Black children averaged ~ 4 hours of screen time/day, Hispanic/Latinx children spent ~ 3 hours of screen time/day, compared with White children who spent ~ 2 hours of screen time/day [3]. Similarly, children from lower income families averaged ~ 4 hours of screen time/day compared with ~ 2 hours of screen time/day in children from higher income families [3]. Yet, digital inequities were exacerbated by the pandemic. As of 2020, 87% of Americans said the Internet was important to them during the outbreak and 53% viewed the Internet as "essential" [4]. Sixty percent of lower income parents reported their children would face at least one digital obstacle schooling from home during the outbreak [5].

Technology use among children and teens continues to be a confusing and heavily debated subject. It is well documented that not all screen time is created equal and it is important to focus on who, how, and what technologies are being used [6,7]. The purpose of this article is to provide a broad overview of technologies commonly used by children and teens and highlight best practices to support safe technology use and positive health outcomes. To help guide our readers, Table 1 provides a summary of common technologies and related terms (at the time of press) used in this article.

HARMS OF TECHNOLOGY USE AMONG CHILDREN, TEENS, AND FAMILIES

Duration of technology use, miscommunication, bullying, unrealistic comparisons, and fear of missing out are contributing factors to low psychological well-being among children and adolescent users of social media [8,9]. In the past, television viewing was nicknamed a "super-peer," suggesting this activity had the same or greater ability to influence children and teens, similar to their peers [10]. Today, a similar label exists for social media "influencers" or individuals capable of shaping decisions of others based on their recognition as an expert or authority [11]. Yet, children and teens developmentally susceptible to feelings and desires, wanting to be "normal," are particularly vulnerable to

Table 1
Common technology terms and examples used among children and teens

Term	Definition	Example
Social media	Web sites and applications that enable users to create and share content or to participate in social networking	TikTok is an app where users can create, watch, and share short-form videos (15–60 s), typically on a smartphone
Smartphone	A mobile phone that performs many of the functions of a computer (eg, touchscreen, Internet, operating systems)	Apple iPhone, Samsung Galaxy, Google Pixel
App	An application downloaded by a user to a mobile device	The Calm App is a health and wellness app that features breathing techniques, calming exercises, and sleep stories to help users practice mindfulness
Screen time	The amount of time an individual spends watching a "screen" typically of a smartphone, tablet, computer, or television	There are parental monitoring apps that can be downloaded to keep track of a person's screen time
Influencer	Individual accounts on social media platforms who have a steady audience and use their account to promote various content	Ryan's World started as a YouTube channel where its influencer, Ryan, shared videos of himself playing with toys, games, and other kid-friendly content
Vlog	Video blog	Addison Rae is a TikTok influencer who shares videos of her dancing
Unboxing	An act or instance of removing a newly purchased product from its packaging and examining its features	Fun toys Collector Disney Toys Review is an unboxing account that opens new toys and dolls from various large companies such as Disney, Pixar, and Nickelodeon
Challenge	A call to record yourself doing some sort of action to share on social media	Devious lick or #deviouslick is where an individual records themselves stealing or destroying items in schools, such as stealing soap dispensers or clogging toilets
Doom scrolling	Continuously scrolling online through bad news	An adolescent who continues to read bad news on twitter may begin to feel like the world is bad
Video chatting	A face-to-face conversation held over the Internet by means of webcams and dedicated software	FaceTime, Google Duo, Zoom, Skype, Discord, Snapchat

(continued on next page)

Table 1 (continued)		
Term	Definition	Example
Multiplayer video games	When more than one person plays the same video game together, either in-person or online	Fortnight, Minecraft, PUBG
Messaging apps	An application where users communicate instantaneously via text messages or emojis	Snap Chat, Kik, WhatsApp, Telegram, GroupMe

photoshopped images or portrayals of altered realities presented as "real." As such, online platforms have been associated with self-esteem issues, bullying, and parenting challenges.

Self-esteem and Technology

Children and teens are prone to compare their own self-image and life to that as presented by others online. Children and teens may try to emulate images, often unrealistic, portrayed by the media and on social media. Social media can be filled with photoshopped and heavily altered pictures and videos, particularly among apps that have filters designed or integrated into the process for posting content. Problems arise when individuals compare their actual self with altered images online, which can be associated with self-esteem [12]. Some research has examined the type of social media use with self-esteem. For example, when teens use social media to post or share their own content, this is described as self-oriented social media use [13]. For teens who use social media this way, a significant amount of time is spent preoccupied over the content they share and peer approval gauged by the number of "likes" [14]. Although viewing positive comments and counting likes can lead to a boost in self-esteem boost, the effect is likely short lived [15]. Conversely, when teens passively view or "like" and comment on the posts of others, this has been described as other-oriented social media. Evidence has shown other-orientated social media use has been linked to decreased self-esteem [13]. In other words, preteen girls who simply looked or commented on others posts, without posting themselves, had lower self-esteem. Facebook's internal research gained national attention in October 2021, when it was suggested that the company ignored data showing that teen girls' thoughts of suicide and eating disorders worsened from Instagram use [16].

Cyberbullying

Cyberbullying is recognized as a dangerous and negative aspect of technology use. Cyberbullying is defined as "willful and repeated harm inflicted through aggressive actions through the use of computers, cell phones, and other electronic devices" [17]. Cyberbullying has been linked to many adverse mental health outcomes, such as depression and suicidal ideation [18,19]. There have been multiple debates as to whether cyberbullying is different or more

Table 2
Exemplar technology resources for providers and parents

Resources for Providers/Parents	Description	Web Site
American Academy of Pediatrics (AAP) Healthy Children Media Page	Healthy Children is the online magazine published by the AAP. It includes a section on media, with many tips for parents and providers on various technology- and media-related concerns. Family Media Use Plan Web site	https://healthychildren .org/english/family-life/media/pages/ default.aspx https://www.healthy children.org/English/ media/Pages/ default.aspx
Common sense media	An independent, nonprofit and research-backed organization that offers parents and schools tips on technology in kids. Movies, shows, books, apps, and video games are rated and reviewed by both experts, other parents, and kids. They also have a K12 Digital Citizens Curriculum	https://www. commonsens emedia.org/
Instagram Parent's Guide	A guidebook put together by Instagram to help parents understand Instagram with safety features, glossary of Instagram terms, and conversation starters	https://about. instagram.com/ community/parents
Joan Ganz Cooney Center	An independent research and innovation laboratory focused on the challenges of educating children in a rapidly changing media landscape whose mission is to advance children's learning through digital media	https://joanganzcoon eycenter.org/
Sesame Street in Communities	Hundreds of bilingual multimedia tools to help kids (age, 6 y) and families expand their knowledge; resources engage kids and adults in daily routines—from teaching early math and literacy concepts, to encouraging families to eat nutritious foods, to serious topics such as divorce and food insecurity	https://sesamestreetin communities.org/

(continued on next page)

Table 2
(continued)

Resources for Providers/Parents	Description	Web Site
One Mind PsyberGuide	Repository of mental health apps that have been rigorously evaluated to improve access to mental health resources	https://onemindpsy berguide.org/ about-psyberguide/
Wait Until 8th	Wait until 8th is a movement focused on helping parents wait until 8th grade to give their kids a cell phone. They also have many resources, such as family guides, app safety, and parent controls	https://www. waituntil8th.org/

harmful than traditional bullying, but often, cyberbullying is seen as an extension of bullying that happens in-person (usually at school). Significant challenges to mitigate cyberbullying include the following: events occur in unmonitored online settings (opposed to school settings), can occur 24/7 (opposed to only during school hours), and can be done by an anonymous user (opposed to known offender) [17]. Furthermore, individuals tend to say things online that they would never say to a person's face, a phenomenon known as online disinhibition [20]. Online disinhibition can be particularly tricky for adolescents and young adults, who already face impulse control issues due to immaturity and an underdeveloped frontal lobe [21].

Parenting Challenges
Nearly 25% of parents say raising kids today is harder than it was 20 years ago, citing technology and social media as the main reasons [22]. Parents are subject to social, peer, and child pressures related to technology. Specific parenting challenges related to technology include, but are not limited to, role-modeling healthy technology behaviors, remaining current about technology trends, keeping their children safe online, and providing (including being able to afford) the right tools so their children can access necessary information for life and school. Nearly 70% of parents report they are sometimes distracted by their phone when they are also with their child, and 50% of parents admit they use their smartphones too much [23]. Numerous parenting blogs and social media sites highlight instances where parents use technology to "babysit" their child or preoccupy their child (ie, to do housework, grocery shop) or keep a child quiet and distracted (eg, at a restaurant). Despite numerous parents and parenting blogs validating technology as a tool for

parenting respite, public sentiment and feedback highlight parental feelings of guilt and shame related to child technology use.

BENEFITS OF TECHNOLOGY USE AMONG CHILDREN, TEENS, AND FAMILIES

Joint Media Engagement

Vital across development, coregulation is the supportive process between adult caregivers and children that fosters the development of self-regulation in children [24]. A child's capacity for self-regulation can dramatically increase during early childhood and adolescents due to changes in brain development [24]. Coregulation consists of the child, the child's relationships, and the child's environment. Technology that jointly engages both the parent and the child can be leveraged during this time to support optimal development. For example, adult caregivers are encouraged to use technology with children, as engagement with both technology and caring adults has been shown to scaffold a child's learning [25]. Previously described as coviewing, joint media engagement refers to both spontaneous and designed experiences for people to engage and use media together [26].

Both before and during the pandemic, social media served as an outlet to marginalized populations (eg, lesbian, gay, bisexual, transgender, and queer) seeking social support, affirmation, and resources [27,28]. During the pandemic, teens quarantined at home went online as a means to independence, connecting with friends and trying new hobbies [29]. Parents can foster their child's growth and development by allowing them developmentally appropriate freedom and privacy, to include going online, which can provide children and teens opportunities to demonstrate capabilities and build confidence.

Tailored and Precision Health

Health care is being transformed by technology with uncharted opportunities for tailored and precision medicine [30]. Several systematic reviews describe the literature on mobile apps used to support behavior change, manage chronic disease, and promote stress management and positive mental health [27,31,32]. There is support for public-private partnerships and repurposing "popular" apps, as stress management interventions have a beneficial impact on reducing stress associated with personal vulnerability, significantly improving overall well-being [30,33]. Across platforms (eg, Apple iOS, Google Play), stress-related apps most frequently used "mindfulness or meditation" or "breathing" exercises [33]. Most of the research indicates positive short-term effects, high patient satisfaction, and unique opportunities to extend health promotion beyond the clinical setting into everyday life.

THE POTENTIAL FOR TECHNOLOGY AMONG CHILDREN, TEENS, AND FAMILIES

Implications for Practice

Parents and children want reliable resources for technology. More than half (61%) of parents say they go to health care providers for advice on technology use in kids [22]. Implicit bias is one area clinicians should strongly reflect on to support technology use among children, teens, and families. Defaulting to a mindset where time spent on technology is "bad" or detrimental reaffirms implicit biases and perpetuates family struggles around technology use. Similarly, it is important that providers recognize technology use between children and parents is interrelated, influenced by parenting style, parent role-modeling, and joint engagement [25,26,34]. Before counseling on technology use, providers should consider real-world perspective of both parents and children. At some point, parents are likely to experience feelings of guilt related to how they themselves use technology or allow their child to use technology. Similarly, many teens will not tell adults when they are experiencing cyberbullying feeling ashamed and for fear that the adult will take away their electronic device [35].

Providers can promote positive parenting by discussing risks and benefits of technology to help guide families. Providers can temper clinical guidelines by focusing on child development and discussing quality of technology use. For example, younger children may not be able to differentiate what is real versus what is fiction. Yet, in older children, filters can be a fun way to express emotions and be creative. Adolescents, who recognize they are exposed to filtered videos and photos on social media have become advocates, prompting hashtags such as #instagramvsreality and #expectationvsreality. Before downloading an app, providers can encourage families to consider the following: (1) does it connect different experiences, (2) does it allow the child to grow and learn, (3) does it encourage communication [36]? If providers are interested in vetting apps before recommending to patients, the uMARS (Mobile Application Rating Scale) is a simple, reliable tool that nondigital health experts can use to assess the quality of apps focused on engagement, aesthetics, information, and functionality [37]. Table 2 also provides a list of exemplar resources for providers and parents.

Several organizations have released guidelines or policy statements on technology use and kids. In 2016, the American Academy of Pediatrics (AAP) Council on Communications and Media published technical reports focused on technology use by age groups and by types of screen time activities [38]. AAP guidelines for media use are highlighted in Table 3. One tool created by AAP to help families navigate technology use among kids is the Family Media Use Plan. This free online tool can be accessed by families in both English and Spanish. A Family Media Use Plan is a plan jointly created with input from all parties involved and may help to improve communication among family members and reduce potential for risky Internet behaviors. The parent may customize the plan for their family as a whole and/or for each child. Some of the specifiers include (1) screen free zones, (2), screen free times (3) device curfews (4) recreational screen time activities, and (5) tips for being a good digital citizen. Among older children and teens, efforts to reduce cyberbullying, either as the bully or the victim, may also benefit from a Family Media Use Plan. Adolescents who report more parental monitoring and efforts to regulate Internet use were less likely to experience cyberbullying compared with those teens who reported less parental

Table 3
Summary of guidelines of technology and social media use in kids by the American Academy of Pediatrics

	The American Academy of Pediatrics
0–2 y	• Prioritize unplugged playtime for infants and toddlers • Avoid screen time other than video-chat for children younger than 18 mo • When introducing media around 18 mo ensure it is high quality and educationally focused (PBS and Sesame Street) • Cowatch media with your child to help them understand what is happening
2–5 y	• Limit screen time to 1 h/d of high-quality programs • No screens during meals or 1 h before bedtime • High-quality children's programming can improve cognitive, literacy, and social outcomes in preschoolers, but parents should be leery, as some programs tout themselves as educational but have no evidence of their efficacy or input from developmental educators • Social skills such as emotional regulation, impulse control, and flexible thinking are still best taught through unstructured and social play • Cowatch media with your child to help them understand what is happening • Parent media use correlates to later child media use. Help parents to take media breaks
6–18 y	• Help children and parents appreciate the good and bad of technology and social media • Create balance between media time and other health behaviors (play, exercise, healthy eating, and sleep) • Place consistent limits on the time spent on screens and the types of content viewed on screens. Family media plans and contracts can help! • Cyberbullying can be very harmful, as it can be anonymous, done 24/7, and spread quickly. Just as children need help navigating in-person adverse peer experiences, they need supportive adult assistance in navigating relationships online • Adolescents vary in their understanding of privacy and the Internet and often need further education

General Tips	• Create a personalized Family Media Plan (available in English and Spanish) https://www.healthychildren.org/English/media/Pages/default.aspx
	• Parents can be "media mentors" teaching their kids digital citizenship
	• There is a correlation between heavy media use and obesity
	   ○ Through a combination of inactivity, commercials about food, and high-caloric snacking in front of screens
	• There is a correlation between heavy media use and sleep issues
	   ○ Through late evening light/screens in bedrooms and suppression of melatonin from blue light
	• There is a correlation between heavy media use and poorer cognitive, language, and social/emotional development across all pediatric ages
	   ○ Through limiting offline relationships, preoccupation with media use over other activities, and multitasking while using media
	• More research needs to be done to understand the relationship between these correlations, but in general keep TVs out of bedrooms and limit screens and social media before bedtime

monitoring [35]. Specifically, regulating Internet time and content, not simply restricting the use of the Internet, was found to be important [35].

Providers should help parents problem solve and provide brainstorm strategies for how to navigate technology and media use in children and teens that best align with real-world expectations. To do this, providers are encouraged to discuss underlying principles of the technology. For example, are the sites the child is using focused on learning something new, communicating with friends, or for entertainment? Can the online activities be substituted or supplemented with an in-person activity? Can the activity be moved to a television or game where the family can enjoy the activity together?

Lastly, providers are encouraged to use general terms (eg, "social media") opposed to specific terms (eg, "TikTok" "Snap Chat") when discussing technology. This strategy is advantageous for 2 reasons: (1) it is not subject to the rapid changes in technology; (2) it can help a clinician maintain credibility, as there are substantial age-related and racial/ethnic differences in platform use. For example, a clinician may ask families what technologies they use to connect with others rather than assume. Nearly half (46%) of Hispanics use the messaging app, "WhatsApp," compared with only 23% of Blacks and 16% of Whites [2]. A clinician may lose or gain credibility if inquiring about a specific platform. Facebook may be one of the most widely used platforms online among American adults (69%), but teens are quickly abandoning Facebook [39]. A clinician would likely fare better by asking, "do you use any social media?" "What is your favorite app?" General questions are likely to spark a conversation and allow the clinician to stay relevant without additional efforts to identify the latest trends.

CLINICS CARE POINTS

- Children, teens, and families continue to use and adopt various technologies making this a critically important topic for health supervision.
- Parents and children look to health care providers for reliable technology-based guidance and resources to foster health and well-being.
- Expert guidelines need to be reconciled with real-world technology use, recognizing that technology use among children and parents is interrelated, and there are both benefits and risks to technology use.
- Providers can temper clinical guidelines by focusing on child development and discussing quality of technology use.
- Implicit bias is one area clinicians can improve to support technology use among children and families, recognizing that not all technology is "bad" and that discussions focused on quality over quantity may lead to productive conversations with families.

SUMMARY

Health care providers should begin conversations regarding technology and family beginning at birth and continuing through adulthood given the omnipresent nature of technology and inevitable exposure [38]. The authors present an overview of technology use among children, teens, and family from both positive and negative perspectives along with broad recommendations. A limitation of this paper is that the technology broadly presented across children and teens. However, we recognize that there is substantial information to present each technology further in-depth, which is beyond the scope of this paper. Furthermore, the authors did not address specific aspects of ethical design, development, and policies (eg, Children's Online Privacy Protection Rule, COPPA) regarding child online safety. The goal of this paper is to support best practices for clinicians who want to help families navigate the ever-changing technology landscape.

DISCLOSURE
The authors report no financial interests or potential conflicts of interest.

References
[1] Anderson M, Jiang J. Teens, Social Media & Technology 2018. Pew Research Center: Internet, Science & Tech. 2018. Available at: http://www.pewinternet.org/2018/05/31/teens-social-media-technology-2018/.

[2] Auxier B, Anderson M. Social Media Use in 2021. Pew Research Center: Internet, Science & Tech. 2021. Available at: https://www.pewresearch.org/internet/2021/04/07/social-media-use-in-2021/.

[3] Rideout V, Robb M. The Common Sense census: media use by kids age zero to eight, 2020. San Francisco, CA: Common Sense Media. 2020. Available at: https://www.commonsensemedia.org/sites/default/files/uploads/research/2020_zero_to_eight_census_final_web.pdf.

[4] Auxier B. How Americans view tech in the time of COVID-19. Pew Research Center. 2020. Available at: https://www.pewresearch.org/fact-tank/2020/12/18/what-weve-learned-about-americans-views-of-technology-during-the-time-of-covid-19/.

[5] Auxier B, Anderson M. As schools close due to the coronavirus, some U.S. students face a digital 'homework gap.' Pew Research Center. 2020. Available at: https://www.pewresearch.org/fact-tank/2020/03/16/as-schools-close-due-to-the-coronavirus-some-u-s-students-face-a-digital-homework-gap/.

[6] Rideout VJ, Katz VS. Opportunity for all? Technology and learning in lower-income families. A report of the Families and Media Project. New York, NY: The Joan Ganz Cooney Center at Sesame Street; 2016.

[7] Orben A, Przybylski AK. The association between adolescent well-being and digital technology use. Nat Hum Behav 2019;3(2):173; https://doi.org/10.1038/s41562-018-0506-1.

[8] Twenge JM, Campbell WK. Media Use Is Linked to Lower Psychological Well-Being: Evidence from Three Datasets. The Psychiatr Q 2019;90(2):311–31; https://doi.org/10.1007/s11126-019-09630-7.

[9] Bloemen N, De Coninck D. Social Media and Fear of Missing Out in Adolescents: The Role of Family Characteristics. Social Media Soc 2020;6(4); https://doi.org/10.1177/2056305120965517:2056305120965517.

[10] Strasburger VC, Wilson BJ, Jordan A. Children, adolescents and the media. Thousand Oaks, CA: Sage Publications; 2008.

[11] Geyser W. What is an Influencer? - Social Media Influencers Defined [Updated 2021]. Influencer Marketing Hub. 2021. Available at: https://influencermarketinghub.com/what-is-an-influencer/.

[12] Vogel E, Rose J, Roberts L, et al. Social comparison, social media, and self-esteem. Psychology of Popular Media Culture. 2014. https://doi.org/10.1037/ppm0000047.

[13] Steinsbekk S, Wichstrøm L, Stenseng F, et al. The impact of social media use on appearance self-esteem from childhood to adolescence – A 3-wave community study. Comp Hum Behav 2021; https://doi.org/10.1016/j.chb.2020.106528.

[14] Yau JC, Reich SM. "It's Just a Lot of Work": Adolescents' Self-Presentation Norms and Practices on Facebook and Instagram. J Res Adolescence 2019; https://doi.org/10.1111/jora.12376.

[15] Krause H-V, Baum K, Baumann A, et al. Unifying the detrimental and beneficial effects of social network site use on self-esteem: a systematic literature review. Media Psychology. 2021. https://doi.org/10.1080/15213269.2019.1656646.

[16] Keith M. Facebook's internal research found its Instagram platform contributes to eating disorders and suicidal thoughts in teenage girls, whistleblower says. Business Insider. 2021. Available at: https://www.businessinsider.com/facebook-knows-data-instagram-eating-disorders-suicidal-thoughts-whistleblower-2021-10. Accessed October 8, 2021.

[17] Hutson E. Cyberbullying in Adolescence: A Concept Analysis. ANS Adv Nurs Sci 2016;39(1):60–70; https://doi.org/10.1097/ANS.0000000000000104.

[18] Bottino SMB, Bottino CMC, Regina CG, et al. Cyberbullying and adolescent mental health: systematic review. Cadernos De Saude Publica 2015;31(3):463–75; https://doi.org/10.1590/0102-311x00036114.

[19] Kwan I, Dickson K, Richardson M, et al. Cyberbullying and Children and Young People's Mental Health: A Systematic Map of Systematic Reviews. Cyberpsychol, Behav Soc Netw 2020; https://doi.org/10.1089/cyber.2019.0370.

[20] Wright MF, Harper BD, Wachs S. The associations between cyberbullying and callous-unemotional traits among adolescents: The moderating effect of online disinhibition. Pers Individ Dif 2019; https://doi.org/10.1016/j.paid.2018.04.001.

[21] Arain M, Haque M, Johal L, et al. Maturation of the adolescent brain. Neuropsychiatr Dis Treat 2013; https://doi.org/10.2147/NDT.S39776.

[22] Auxier B, Anderson M, Perrin A, et al. Parenting Children in the Age of Screens. Pew Research Center: Internet. Sci Tech 2020. Available at: https://www.pewresearch.org/internet/2020/07/28/parenting-children-in-the-age-of-screens/.

[23] Anderson M. How parents feel about – and manage – their teens' online behavior and screen time. Pew Research Center. 2019. Available at: https://www.pewresearch.org/fact-tank/2019/03/22/how-parents-feel-about-and-manage-their-teens-online-behavior-and-screen-time/.

[24] Rosanbalm, K. D., & Murray, D. W. (2017). Caregiver Co-regulation Across Development: A Practice Brief. (No. OPRE Brief #2017-80). Washington, D.C.: Office of Planning, Research and Evaluation, Administration for Children and Families, U.S. Department of Health and Human Services.

[25] Zack E, Barr R. The Role of Interactional Quality in Learning from Touch Screens during Infancy: Context Matters. Front Psychol 2016;7:1264; https://doi.org/10.3389/fpsyg.2016.01264.

[26] Takeuchi L, Stevens R. The New Coviewing: designing for learning through joint media engagement. 2011. Available at: http://joanganzcooneycenter.org/publication/the-new-coviewing-designing-for-learning-through-joint-media-engagement/.

[27] Escobar-Viera CG, Melcher EM, Miller RS, et al. A systematic review of the engagement with social media–delivered interventions for improving health outcomes among sexual and gender minorities. Internet Interventions 2021;25:100428; https://doi.org/10.1016/j.invent.2021.100428.

[28] Harper GW, Serrano PA, Bruce D, et al. The Internet's Multiple Roles in Facilitating the Sexual Orientation Identity Development of Gay and Bisexual Male Adolescents. Am J Men's Health 2016;10(5):359–76; https://doi.org/10.1177/1557988314566227.

[29] Dennen VP, Rutledge SA, Bagdy LM, et al. Virtual Independence: Teen Social Media Use During the Summer of Quarantine. 2021. Available at: https://www.ict-conf.org/wp-content/uploads/2021/07/03_202106C028_Dennen.pdf.

[30] Arigo D, Jake-Schoffman DE, Wolin K, et al. The history and future of digital health in the field of behavioral medicine. J Behav Med 2019;42(1):67–83; https://doi.org/10.1007/s10865-018-9966-z.

[31] Hale K, Capra S, Bauer J. A Framework to Assist Health Professionals in Recommending High-Quality Apps for Supporting Chronic Disease Self-Management: Illustrative Assessment of Type 2 Diabetes Apps. JMIR mHealth and uHealth 2015;3(3):e4532; https://doi.org/10.2196/mhealth.4532.

[32] Rathbone AL, Clarry L, Prescott J. Assessing the Efficacy of Mobile Health Apps Using the Basic Principles of Cognitive Behavioral Therapy: Systematic Review. J Med Internet Res 2017;19(11):e399; https://doi.org/10.2196/jmir.8598.

[33] Lau N, O'Daffer A, Colt S, et al. Android and iPhone Mobile Apps for Psychosocial Wellness and Stress Management: Systematic Search in App Stores and Literature Review. JMIR mHealth and uHealth 2020;8(5):e17798; https://doi.org/10.2196/17798.

[34] Pina LR, Sien S-W, Ward T, et al. From Personal Informatics to Family Informatics: Understanding Family Practices Around Health Monitoring. In: Proceedings of the 2017 ACM Conference on computer supported Cooperative Work and social computing. Portland, OR, USA: ACM; 2017. p. 2300–15; https://doi.org/10.1145/2998181.2998362, Presented at the CSCW.

[35] Fenaughty J, Harré N. Factors associated with young people's successful resolution of distressing electronic harassment. Comput Education 2013;61:242–50; https://doi.org/10.1016/j.compedu.2012.08.004.

[36] Gee E, Takeuchi L, Wartella E, editors. Children and families in the digital age: learning together in a media Saturated Culture (Paperback) - Routledge. New York, NY, USA: Taylor & Francis; 2018. Available at: https://www.routledge.com/Children-and-Families-in-the-Digital-Age-Learning-Together-in-a-Media/Gee-Takeuchi-Wartella/p/book/9781138238619.

[37] Stoyanov SR, Hides L, Kavanagh DJ, et al. Development and Validation of the User Version of the Mobile Application Rating Scale (uMARS). JMIR mHealth and uHealth 2016;4(2):e72; https://doi.org/10.2196/mhealth.5849.

[38] Chassiakos Y, Linda) R, Radesky J, et al. Children and Adolescents and Digital Media. Pediatrics 2016;138(5); https://doi.org/10.1542/peds.2016-2593.

[39] Perrin A, Anderson M. Share of U.S. adults using social media, including Facebook, is mostly unchanged since 2018. Pew Research Center. 2019. Available at: https://www.pewresearch.org/fact-tank/2019/04/10/share-of-u-s-adults-using-social-media-including-facebook-is-mostly-unchanged-since-2018/.

Treating Adolescent Anxiety and Depression in Primary Care Considering Pandemic Mental Health Fallout

Michele Davide, MS, APN, FNP-BC

Advocare West Morris Pediatrics, 151 Route 10 East, Suite 105, Succasunna, NJ 07876, USA

Keywords

- Adolescent • Depression • Anxiety • Evidence-based • Interventions
- Mental health • Primary care • Pandemic

Key points

- A longstanding, worsening epidemic of adolescent depression and anxiety was made significantly worse by the COVID-19 Pandemic, causing functional impairment in teens and caregiver strain.
- Published evidence-based guidelines and toolkits to treat adolescent depression and anxiety are not being routinely implemented in pediatric primary care practices.
- Pediatric primary care practitioners must embrace adolescent mental wellness and make practice changes to meet the needs of their patients and fill in mental health treatment gaps.
- Pediatric primary care practitioners must identify and break down barriers to mental health treatment and commit to help combat the National Children's Mental Health Emergency.
- Pediatric primary care practitioners must advocate for policies, programs, and funding to improve the mental health of their patients.

OVERVIEW

Pediatric mental health describes the emotional, cognitive, and social well-being of children, as reflected by the achievement of developmental milestones, formation of relationships, and ability to cope with adversity. Pediatric mental illness occurs when children are unable to think, act, and feel in an

E-mail address: midavide16@gmail.com

https://doi.org/10.1016/j.yfpn.2021.12.015
2589-420X/22/© 2022 Elsevier Inc. All rights reserved.

age-appropriate manner, which interferes with functioning at home, school, and in social settings [1].

Mental health challenges are common in children and adolescents, affecting up to 20% of the pediatric population, and are often unrecognized and untreated [2–8]. The prevalence of anxiety and depression increases with age from childhood into adolescence [8], and the rates of each disorder have been increasing. In 2009, 26.9% of high school students experienced persistent sadness or hopelessness and that rate increased to 36.7% in 2019. The lifetime prevalence of adolescent anxiety is 31.9% with 8.3% experiencing severe impairment [5]. The reported prevalence of pediatric mental health disorders is likely underrepresented since children and parents are often unwilling to report mental health concerns or unaware that their symptoms are treatable [5,9].

The National Association of Pediatric Nurse Practitioners (NAPNAP), the American Academy of Pediatrics (AAP), and the American Board of Pediatrics (ABP) prioritized integrating emotional and behavioral assessment and treatment into routine pediatric care as a strategy to help solve the youth mental health provider shortage [10–12].

Beginning in March of 2020, COVID-19 pandemic-induced stressors intensified an underlying epidemic of underrecognized and undertreated pediatric mental illness and brought it into the spotlight [13]. Uncertainty, loss, isolation, disruptions to social connections, and restricted access to school-based resources led to widespread fear and sadness [14]. Global disruptions and challenges caused by the pandemic created "an overall strain on hope, resilience, and perseverance." [15] Reports of increased pediatric emergency room visits and boarding for psychiatric complaints including suicidality gained national attention and a call to action [14,16–19]. The increase in pediatric mental illness led to the declaration of "A National Emergency in Children's Mental Health" by children's health advocacy organizations on October 19, 2021 [20].

The pandemic raised awareness that adverse childhood events and social determinants of health (SDOH) lead to poor mental and physical health outcomes [13,21–23], and underscored the importance of providing trauma-informed care and early identification and treatment of mental health challenges [14,23].

Stressful events are known to trigger behavioral reactions in children and adolescents [15]. Isolation and loneliness, two known risk factors for pediatric depression and anxiety, were ubiquitous during pandemic lockdowns [24]. Adolescents as a group were severely affected by the COVID-19 crisis, which resulted in increased fear, sadness, aggression, irritability, and substance use [14,15].

Studies showed that during the first few months of the COVID-19 pandemic, a quarter of high school students reported a decline in mental health, and several months later only 33% of high school students "were able to cope with their sources of stress, which include strained mental health and peer relationships." [24].

The COVID-19 Pandemic created an opportunity to destigmatize mental health through a universal experience of depression and anxiety [25]. Pandemic relief funds were allocated to address the pediatric mental health crisis and dismantle barriers to mental health care through awareness, education, tele-health, and collaboration initiatives [26,27]. The goal of these programs is to overcome logistical and financial barriers to care (Fig. 1) and reduce the stigma of mental illness [27]. Despite research disproving myths and the high preva-lence of mental illness, stigma remains one of the most difficult barriers to over-come, hindering the identification and treatment of mental health disorders [28–30]. Improving the proficiency of pediatric primary care providers treating mental illness will require identifying and overcoming barriers, practice prepa-ration, training, and coordination, and the process will be different for every practitioner [10,12,31].

Components of impactful and evidence-based practice improvements include (Fig. 2)

- Needs assessment
- Staff education
- Mental health emergency plan
- Increased screening
- Collaboration
- Interventions
- Follow-up
- Practitioner education
- Advocacy

NEEDS ASSESSMENT

Each practitioner should take an inventory of their strengths and weaknesses, and recognize barriers they face that interfere with their ability to confidently treat mental health concerns [12,31]. The AAP published a Mental Health Toolkit in 2021 which includes a comprehensive Mental Health Practice

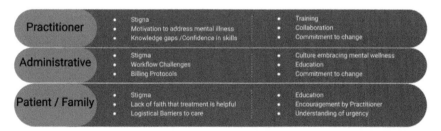

Fig. 1. Barriers to care and opportunities for improvement. (*Data from* Green CM, Foy JM, Earls MF and Committee on Psychosocial Aspects of Child and Family Health, Mental Health Leadership Work Group. Achieving the Pediatric Mental Health Competencies. Pediatrics. 2019;144(5) doi https://doi.org/10.1542/peds.2019-2758; and Marian F. Earls MF, Foy JM, Green CM. Mental health toolkit addressing mental health concerns in pediatrics: a prac-tical resource toolkit for clinicians, 2nd Edition. Itasca, IL. American Academy of Pediatrics; 2021).

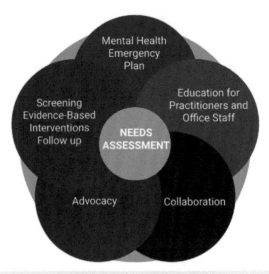

Fig. 2. Key Components of the Primary Care Workflow to improve mental health practice. (*Data from* Refs [10,12,15,31–38,41,42]).

Readiness Inventory for providers who are interested in transforming their practice to better meet the mental health care needs of their patients [31].

STAFF EDUCATION

Throughout the COVID-19 pandemic, everyone including parents, children, staff members, and providers experienced unprecedented stress [32]. Pediatric primary care offices should be safe spaces where employees understand their role in supporting the mental health of the youth they serve. Practitioners should encourage self-care techniques for their staff, increase awareness about the importance of mental health, and inspire a cultural transformation to become a practice that embraces mental wellness [10,12,31–38].

Using a crisis lens, pediatric office staff should routinely ask parents how they are coping with stress [39]. The nursing and medical staff should incorporate an assessment of signs of mental health challenges and mental wellness counseling into every patient encounter [10,21,32,39]. It is important that the office staff is involved in planning new protocols, understands the importance of proposed interventions, and is adequately trained before the implementation of new procedures to prevent the frustration and resentment that frequently accompany change [40].

MENTAL HEALTH EMERGENCY PLAN

There should be a mental health emergency plan in place in the event that a patient reports suicidal ideation [31,41]. Patients must be assessed and referred appropriately, by contacting 911, the mobile response team, the suicide phone or text number or a community mental health specialist. Practitioners must be comfortable addressing suicide safety planning, including counseling on restricting access to lethal means, warning signs, and educating youth and caregivers about the importance of at-risk patients engaging with a trusted adult [31,41]. Practitioners should frequently follow-up with at-risk patients to build and maintain a therapeutic relationship and serially assess changes in risk [3,31,41]. The AAP mental health toolkit includes a Practice Preparations and Triage for Psychiatric Emergencies worksheet to help offices prepare for psychiatric emergencies [31].

SCREENING

Mental health screening should take place at every well, sick, and follow-up visit due to the increased incidence of mental distress [12]. (Fig. 3) Framing mental wellness as a continuum instead of focusing on diagnosing mental health disorders may normalize the conversation and help patients and practitioners overcome negative thoughts and feelings associated with mental illness [25,29,30,42]. In addition to mental health screening, providers should screen for adverse childhood experiences (ACES) and SDOH with validated tools [13]. Early identification and management of mental health symptoms will help patients and families avoid long-term consequences of untreated mental illness, and alleviate the ripple effect of untreated mental illness including lost productivity and strain on caregivers [36].

Routine screening is already being conducted at well visits by many practices [43]. Increasing screening to every visit and seamlessly following up positive initial broad symptom screens with symptom-specific screens is a technique that nursing staff can implement so practitioners have a baseline of information prior to starting each patient encounter [31,44].

There are several freely available, evidence-based, validated behavioral screening tools available. For infants and children five and under, age-specific

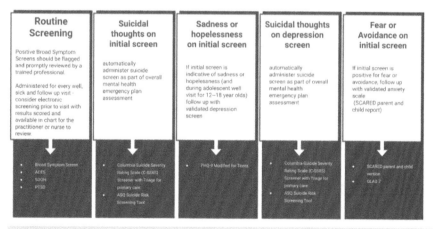

Fig. 3. Approach to increased mental health screening in primary care. (*Data from* Refs [12,15,21,31]).

SWYC screening scales are used to screen for general behavioral and developmental concerns [31,32,45]. For children ages 18 and 24 months, the M-CHAT-R/F autism screening tool is used [32,33,46]. For older children and adolescents, the Pediatric Symptom Checklist is a freely available and validated broad-based screening tool with a parent version for youth 6 to 18 years (PSC-35) and a self-report version for youth 11 to 18 years (PSY-35), and use subscales to look for internalizing, externalizing and behavioral concerns [32,33,47].

When broad-based screening tools are positive, symptom-specific screening tools should be administered. After a broad symptom screen indicates the presence of a depressive disorder, (and during well visits for adolescents ages 12–18) a validated depression screen such as the PHQ-9, modified for adolescents, should be given [32,33,48]. When a depression screen is positive for suicidality, it should be promptly followed by a validated suicide screen such as the Columbia-Suicide Severity Rating Scale (C-SSRS) Screener with triage for primary care settings [12,32,33,49]. When fear and avoidance behaviors are noted on an initial screen, The SCARED screen helps differentiate the severity and classification of anxiety symptoms [32,33,50]. When a patient screens positive for a disorder, the practitioner must interview the patient and family to further explore the severity of symptoms and functional impact and to initiate a plan of care [32,33].

Incorporating formal screening into each patient encounter creates logistical challenges. The AAP offers assistance through the Screening Technical Assistance and Resource (STAR) program to support practitioners establish routine screening procedures [44].

COLLABORATION

Collaborative care initiatives between child and adolescent psychiatrists and pediatric primary care practitioners have been shown to successfully increase access to youth mental health care and improve the competence and confidence of primary care providers in managing mental illness [51–56]. Many states implemented pediatric behavioral health collaboratives, modeled after the successful Massachusetts initiative to encourage pediatric providers to consult and comanage patients with mental health experts [10,51–56]. Pediatric primary care practitioners should participate in collaborative models to improve mental health outcomes [57]. Referral to mental health specialists will always be an essential part of pediatric primary care. In addition to becoming more adept at identifying mental health concerns and managing mild to moderate symptoms, it is essential for pediatric providers to be familiar with specialists in their community and knowledgeable about the specific services they provide.

INTERVENTIONS

In addition to collaborative care models, several other primary care-based interventions have been shown to improve mental health outcomes in pediatrics (Fig. 4). The most robust evidence supports the use of

- Cognitive behavioral therapy (CBT)

Cognitive Behavioral Therapy	Medication Management	Common Factors Approach	Common Elements Approach	Anticipatory Guidance
• Understand basic CBT principles • Refer to mental health specialists in the community who use CBT • Learn and offer CBT as a treatment modality for patients with mild to moderate symptoms. • Hire a mental health specialist to offer CBT. • Consider online, written or app based self-guided CBT designed for parents and teens who are motivated to reduce symptoms of anxiety and depression and improve their function yet are resistant to traditional therapy.	• Complete CME courses on psychopharmacology • Review psychopharmacology guidelines • Participate in collaborative programs where child and adolescent psychiatrists offer consultation and co-management of pediatric patients with mental health concern. • Participate in case based, interactive educational opportunities, such as the AAP Echo Program	• Transdiagnostic communication tool • Hope, empathy, active listening, culturally appropriate language • ask permission to address mental health concerns • partner with the patient and family to create a treatment plan found to be helpful across mental illness concerns	• Symptom specific communication tool • Focuses on symptom clusters • Fear: gradual exposure, distraction, parental role modeling • Sadness: share message of hope, emphasize strengths, review coping mechanisms	• Attachment • Time Ins • Sleep • Nutrition • Exercise • Mindfulness • Meditation • Tense and relax muscles • Quickly share age and symptom specific resources

Fig. 4. Overview of primary care adolescent anxiety and depression interventions. (*Data from* Refs [12,21,28,31]).

- Medication management
- CBT plus medication management [31].

This is a strong evidence-based showing these interventions reduce symptoms of anxiety and depression and improve functioning [31]. Many pediatric practitioners are not comfortable offering these interventions and will require additional training and collaboration prior to routine implementation [57–59].

Basic anticipatory guidance when counseling families about mental wellness during primary care visits should include stressing the importance of the following to protect mental health:

- Attachment
- Time-ins
- Adequate Sleep
- Nutrition
- Exercise [10,12].

It is also important to incorporate the following messages into primary care visits when communicating with children and families about mental health concerns [10,12].

- Protective factors
- Risk factors
- Strengths
- Validation
- Hope
- Reflective Listening
- Follow-up questions
- Mindfulness
- Gratitude
- Meditation
- Relaxation

- Tense/Relax Muscles

The AAP recommends using the evidence-based transdiagnostic Common Factors Approach to communicate with families to facilitate a therapeutic alliance and offer basic elements of therapy shown to be effective for a variety of mental health symptoms. This is a brief intervention focusing on hope, empathy, active listening, culturally appropriate language, asking permission to address mental health concerns, and partnering with the patient and family to create a treatment plan [31]. The AAP created the pnmonic HELP to summarize the components of the Common Factors Approach and recommends using this technique to offer basic psychoeducation across symptoms and to help close a visit and plan follow-up care [31].

The symptom-specific Common Elements Approach is another evidence-based communication tool recommended by the AAP [31]. This tool focuses on symptom clusters such as fear or sadness to guide communication. For anxiety concerns, this technique includes education about anxiety, gradual exposure, distraction techniques, and parental role modeling. For depressive concerns, this includes a message of hope, an inventory of strengths, and a review of coping skills and problem-solving techniques [31].

Evidence-based parenting classes should be discussed with families who struggle to manage children with challenging behaviors. The Triple P and Incredible Years programs are available online and have been shown to be effective at increasing parental competencies and reducing challenging behavior [60–62]. The California evidence-based clearinghouse for child welfare information and resources for child welfare professionals created an online tool for evaluating parenting resources and includes the evidence base as part of the evaluation [63]. This interactive tool is useful for pediatric providers to guide parents who require assistance in building specific skills and overcoming a variety of parenting challenges toward evidence-based courses [63].

Sharing resources such as websites and books that are supported by evidence increases a family's involvement and investment in maximizing their mental wellness. Practitioners should become familiar with resources and have the ability to locate and distribute them during patient visits [12,31,32]. Organizing quick texts and electronic links to resources or a paper-based inventory by age and symptoms is a technique that can save time during visits.

Practitioners should be knowledgeable about online courses that may be useful for families facing mental health challenges. The National Alliance on Mental Illness offers a free 6-part self-guided course for caregivers of children and adolescents showing symptoms of mental illness and has been shown to improve family functioning [64,65]. There are self-directed CBT-based online programs such as My Anxiety Plan for Children and Teens and Creating Opportunities for Personal Empowerment (COPE) available for adolescents who are motivated to decrease their symptoms and impairment [66,67].

Practitioners should educate themselves about digital therapeutics (Dtx) designed to deliver behavioral health treatments through technology devices.

This technology is emerging as a way to potentially increase access to pediatric mental health care, and practitioners should stay current on research and development in this area. There are over 10,000 mobile mental health apps available for download and pediatric patients are using them [68,69]. Pediatric providers are compelled to become familiar with these products and assist their patients in making informed decisions about how to evaluate them [68,69].

The mobile mental health app evaluation tools the APA's APP Advisor and the Mobile App Rating Scale (MARS) enable practitioners to help patients make informed decisions about using these resources [68,69]. The first CBT-based, prescription digital therapeutic product aimed at treating adolescent depression, LIMBIX Spark announced its intention to seek FDA approval at the October 2021 AAP Conference and began negotiating reimbursement rates with insurance companies [70,71].

PRACTITIONER EDUCATION

Pediatric practitioners should seek educational opportunities to increase their competence and confidence in pediatric mental health treatments.

- The *Reach Institute* offers a variety of workshops and a 3-day fellowship program for pediatric providers that teach evidence-based mental health therapies [12,32,72].
- The *Ohio State University's KySS Child and Adolescent Mental Health Online Fellowship* is a program designed to train primary care pediatric providers in treating mental illness. This forum offers twelve online, self-paced modules that outline evidence-based treatments for children and teens facing mental health challenges [12,32,73].
- The *AAP* offers collaborative workshops where pediatric primary care providers and mental health specialists meet over a period of weeks or months and review didactic information about the child and mental health topics and break into small groups to discuss cases. This format allows pediatric providers to learn from each other and increase their comfort level in mental illness identification and treatment.

FOLLOW-UP

Following up with patients who have mental health concerns allows providers to strengthen the therapeutic relationship and track symptom progression over time [31,32]. The AAP Mental Health Care Algorithm recommends that all children with behavioral health concerns or positive screenings should be placed on a practice registry, to be followed over time, and offered trasdiagnotic and symptom-specific treatments within the pediatric practice, which have been shown to help reduce symptoms of mental health disorders in children [37].

ADVOCACY

Pediatric primary care practitioners are natural advocates for pediatric mental healthcare. Advocacy efforts are underway in many areas including but not limited to:

- Collaborative care programs
- Increased funding for pediatric mental health care
- Improved and novel reimbursement arrangements
- Increased mental health training for current and future practitioners
- Programs to reduce the stigma of mental illness
- Streamlined billing policies
- Increased communication between providers [10,12,42].

Involvement with local and national organizations devoted to improving the health of children is a logical first step in advocacy for practitioners who are passionate about children's health [10,12,42].

CONCLUSION

Guidelines from The National Association of Pediatric Nurse Practitioners and the American Academy of Pediatrics stress the importance of focusing on mental health promotion and screening, implementing evidence-based interventions, increasing knowledge of mental health interventions, collaborating, and advocating for essential child mental health elements to be incorporated into pediatric primary care. This requires time, coordination, and commitment. Responding to the National Children's Mental Health Emergency starts with each pediatric practitioner making a change.

As David Satcher, the former U.S. Surgeon General noted in 1999 a statement that remains true today and must be addressed by every pediatric health care provider.

Promoting mental health for all Americans will require scientific know-how but, even more importantly, a societal resolve that we will make the needed investment. The investment does not call for massive budgets; rather, it calls for the willingness of each of us to educate ourselves and others about mental health and mental illness, and thus to confront the attitudes, fear, and misunderstanding that remain as barriers before us [74].

Our nation's children can no longer wait for us to gradually overcome barriers to mental health treatment. Impactful changes must be made now before the crisis worsens. Children's lives are at stake and they are depending on us to protect them.

CLINICS CARE POINTS

- Embrace pediatric mental health.
- Implement screening for pediatric mental health concerns during every patient encounter.
- Increase knowledge of evidence-based pediatric mental health treatments and incorporate them into primary care.
- Collaborate with Child and Adolescent Psychiatrists.
- Advocate for initiatives to support pediatric mental health.

Acknowledgments

The author would like to thank Dr. Stephane Evan's for her guidance and insightful perspectives regarding the role of nurse practitioners in supporting pediatric mental health.

Disclosure

The author has nothing to disclose.

References

[1] What is children's mental health? Centers for Disease Control and Prevention; 2021. Available at: https://www.cdc.gov/childrensmentalhealth/basics.htm. Accessed October 20, 2021.

[2] Perou R, Bitsko RH, Blumberg SJ, et al. Mental health surveillance among children—United States, 2005-2011. MMWR Suppl 2013;62(2):1–35. Available at: https://www.cdc.gov/mmwr/preview/mmwrhtml/su6202a1.htm. Accessed October 20, 2021.

[3] National Research Council (US) and Institute of Medicine (US) Committee on the Prevention of Mental Disorders and Substance Abuse Among Children, Youth, and Young Adults: Research Advances and Promising Interventions. In: O'Connell ME, Boat T, Warner KE, editors. Preventing mental, emotional, and behavioral disorders among young people: progress and possibiliies. National Academies Press (US); 2009. Available at: https://www.ncbi.nlm.nih.gov/books/NBK32788/.

[4] Mental Health. World Health Organization. 2019. Available at: http://www.who.int/features/factfiles/mental_health/en/index.html. Accessed October 20, 2021.

[5] Merikangas KR, He JP, Brody D, et al. Prevalence and treatment of mental disorders among U.S. children in the 2001–2004 NHANES. Pediatrics 2010;125(1):75–81; https://doi.org/10.1542/peds.2008-2598.

[6] NAMI. Mental health by the numbers. Available at: https://www.nami.org/mhstats. Accessed September 20, 2021.

[7] Danielson ML, Bitsko RH, Ghandour RM, et al. Prevalence of parent-reported ADHD diagnosis and associated treatment among U.S. children and adolescents. J Clin Child Adolesc Psychol 2018;47(2):199–212; https://doi.org/10.1080/15374416.2017.1417860.

[8] Ghandour RM, Sherman LJ, Vladutiu CJ, et al. Prevalence and treatment of depression, anxiety, and conduct problems in U.S. children. J Pediatr 2019;206:256–67; https://doi.org/10.1016/j.jpeds.2018.09.021.

[9] Data and statistics on children's mental health. Centers for Disease Control and Prevention; 2021. Available at: https://www.cdc.gov/childrensmentalhealth/data.html. Accessed October 21, 2021.

[10] Frye L, Van Cleve S, Heighway S, et al. NAPNAP position statement on the integration of mental health care in pediatric primary care settings. J Pediatr Health Care 2020;34(5):514–7; https://doi.org/10.1016/j.pedhc.2020.04.013.

[11] McMillan JA, Land M, Leslie LK. Pediatric residency education and the behavioral and mental health crisis: a call to action. Pediatrics 2016;139(1); https://doi.org/10.1542/peds.2016-2141.

[12] Green CM, Foy JM, Earls MF, Committee on Psychosocial Aspects of Child and Family Health, Mental Health Leadership Work Group. Achieving the pediatric mental health competencies. Pediatrics 2019;144(5); https://doi.org/10.1542/peds.2019-2758.

[13] Wyckoff AS. Supporting emotional, behavioral needs of children in the pandemic: updated guidance. Am Acad Pediatr 2021. Available at: https://www.aappublications.org/news/2021/08/02/emotional-behavioral-health-covid-080221. Accessed September 24, 2021.

[14] Meade J. Mental health effects of the covid-19 pandemic on children and adolescents: a review of the current research. Pediatr Clin North Am 2021. Available at: https://pubmed.ncbi.nlm.nih.gov/34538305/. Accessed September 26, 2021.

[15] American Academy of Pediatrics. Interim guidance on supporting the emotional and behavioral health needs of children, adolescents, and families during the COVID-19 Pandemic 2021. Available at: https://www.aap.org/en/pages/2019-novel-coronavirus-covid-19-infections/clinical-guidance/interim-guidance-on-supporting-the-emotional-and-behavioral-health-needs-of-children-adolescents-and-families-during-the-covid-19-pandemic/. Accessed September 21, 2021.

[16] Yard E, Radhakrishnan L, Ballesteros MF, et al. Emergency department visits for suspected suicide attempts among persons aged 12–25 years before and during the COVID-19 Pandemic-United States, January 2019–May 2021. Morb Mortal Wkly Rep 2021;70: 888–94; https://doi.org/10.15585/mmwr.mm7024e1.

[17] Bebinger M. No vacancy: how a shortage of mental health beds in treatment centers keeps teens trapped inside ERs. WBUR News; 2021. Available at: https://www.wbur.org/news/2021/05/17/children-teens-emergency-room-boarding-mental-health. Accessed September 27, 2021.

[18] Hoffman M. Rady Children's seeing 25% increase in mental health ER visits. Kpbs. 2021. Available at: https://www.kpbs.org/news/2021/jun/09/rady-childrens-seeing-25-increase-mental-health-em/. Accessed September 27, 2021.

[19] Stainton LH. Coronavirus pandemic mental health, substance use visits to ER reflect 'a pandemic within a pandemic' in N.J.; greatest toll on the young. WHYY.com; 2021. Available at: https://whyy.org/articles/mental-health-substance-use-visits-to-er-reflect-a-pandemic-within-a-pandemic-in-n-j-greatest-toll-on-the-young/. Accessed September 26, 2021.

[20] American Academy of Pediatrics. AAP, AACAP, CHA declare national emergency in children's mental health. AAP News; 2021. Available at: https://www.aappublications.org/news/2021/10/19/children-mental-health-national-emergency-101921. Accessed October 20, 2021.

[21] Melnyk BM, Jensen P, editors. A practical guide to child and adolescent mental health screening, early intervention, and health promotion. 2nd edition. New York, NY: National Association of Pediatric Nurse Practitioners; 2013.

[22] Bartek N, Peck JL, Garzon D, et al. Addressing the clinical impact of Covid-19 on pediatric mental health. J Pediatr Health Care 2021;35(4):377–86; https://doi.org/10.1016/j.pedhc.2021.03.006.

[23] Adverse Childhood Experiences (ACEs): Preventing Early Trauma to Improve Adult Health. Centers for Disease Control and Prevention; 2019. Available at: https://www.cdc.gov/vitalsigns/aces/. Accessed October 21, 2021.

[24] Panchal N, Kamal R, Cox C, et al. Mental health and substance use considerations among children during the COVID-19 pandemic. KFF (blog); 2021. Available at: https://www.kff.org/coronavirus-covid-19/issue-brief/mental-health-and-substance-use-considerations-among-children-during-the-covid-19-pandemic/. Accessed September 28, 2021.

[25] Gold J. Could COVID-19 finally destigmatize mental illness? Time; 2020. Available at : https://time.com/5835960/coronavirus-mental-illness-stigma/. Accessed September 27, 2021.

[26] BPC Behavioral Health Integration Task Force. Tackling America's mental health and addiction crisis through primary care integration: task force recommendations. Bipartisan Policy Center; 2021. Available at: https://bipartisanpolicy.org/download/?file=/wp-content/uploads/2021/03/BPC_Behavioral-Health-Integration-report_R03.pdf. Accessed September 23, 2021.

[27] Simmons-Duffin S, Chatterjee R. Children's mental health gets millions in funding from the Biden administration. NPR; 2021. Available at: https://www.npr.org/sections/back-to-school-live-updates/2021/08/27/1031493941/childrens-mental-health-gets-millions-in-funding-from-the-biden-administration. Accessed September 23, 2021.

[28] Foy JM, Green CM, Earls MF, Committee on Psychosocial Aspects of Child and Family Health, Mental Health Leadership Work Group. Mental health competencies for pediatric practice. Pediatrics 2019;144(5); https://doi.org/10.1542/peds.2019-2757.

[29] Ahmedani BK. Mental health stigma: society, individuals, and the profession. J Soc Work Values Ethics 2011. Available at: https://www.ncbi.nlm.nih.gov/pmc/articles/PMC3248273/. Accessed September 28, 2021.

[30] Holder SM, Peterson ER, Stephens R, et al. Stigma in mental health at the macro and micro levels: implications for mental health consumers and professionals. Community Ment Health J 2018;55(3):369–74; https://doi.org/10.1007/s10597-018-0308-y.

[31] Marian F, Earls MF, Foy JM, et al. Mental health toolkit addressing mental health concerns in pediatrics: a practical resource toolkit for clinicians. 2nd edition. Itasca, IL: American Academy of Pediatrics; 2021.

[32] Kearney A, Hamel L, Brodie M. Mental health impact of the COVID-19 pandemic: an update. KFF; 2021. Available at: https://www.kff.org/coronavirus-covid-19/poll-finding/mental-health-impact-of-the-covid-19-pandemic. Accessed October 22, 2021.

[33] Zuckerbrot RA, Cheung A, Jensen PS, et al, Glad-PC Steering Group. Guidelines for adolescent depression in primary care (GLAD-PC): part I. Practice preparation, identification, assessment, and initial management. Pediatrics 2018;141(3); https://doi.org/10.1542/peds.2017-4081.

[34] Cheung AH, Zuckerbrot RA, Jensen PS, et al, Glad-PC Steering Group. Guidelines for adolescent depression in primary care (GLAD-PC): part II. Treatment and ongoing management. Pediatrics 2018;141(3); https://doi.org/10.1542/peds.2017-4082.

[35] Monroeac C, Lorestoab F, Horton-Deutschc S, et al. The value of intentional self-care practices: the effects of mindfulness on improving job satisfaction, teamwork, and workplace environments. Arch Psychiatr Nurs 2020;35(2):189–94; https://doi.org/10.1016/j.apnu.2020.10.003.

[36] Whitney DG, Peterson MD. US national and state-level prevalence of mental health disorders and disparities of mental health care use in children. JAMA Pediatr 2019;173(4):389; https://doi.org/10.1001/jamapediatrics.2018.5399. https://time.com/5835960/coronavirus-mental-illness-stigma/.

[37] American Academy of Pediatrics. Mental health care in pediatrics. 2021. Available at: https://downloads.aap.org/AAP/PDF/Algorithm_Integration_of_Mental_Health_Care_Into_Pediatric_Practice.pdf. Accessed October 20, 2021.

[38] American Academy of Pediatrics. Mental health initiatives. 2021. Available at: https://www.aap.org/en/patient-care/mental-health-initiatives/. Accessed October 20, 2021.

[39] Rider EA, Ansari E, Varrin PH, et al. Mental health and wellbeing of children and adolescents during the covid-19 pandemic. BMJ 2021;374; https://doi.org/10.1136/bmj.n1730.

[40] Vosa JFJ, Rupertb J. Change agent's contribution to recipients' resistance to change: A two-sided story. Eur Manag J 2018;36(4):453–62. https://www.sciencedirect.com/science/article/pii/S0263237317301512#.

[41] Treatment for suicidal ideation, self-harm, and suicide attempts among youth. SAMHSA. Available at: https://www.samhsa.gov/resource/ebp/treatment-suicidal-ideation-self-harm-suicide-attempts-among-youth. Accessed September 26, 2021.

[42] Adam D. Mental health: on the spectrum. Nature 2013;496:416–8.

[43] Joseph J, Kagadkar F, Galanter CA. Screening for behavioral health issues in primary care. Curr Treat Options Peds 2018;4:129–45; https://doi.org/10.1007/s40746-018-0118-z.

[44] Screening, Technical Assistance and Resource (STAR) Center. Available at: https://www.aap.org/en/patient-care/screening-technical-assistance-and-resource-center/. Accessed October 21, 2021.

[45] Tufts Medical Center. The survey of well-being of young children. Available at: https://www.tuftschildrenshospital.org/the-survey-of-wellbeing-of-young-children/overview. Accessed October 20, 2021.

[46] Robins DL. M-CHAT™. Available at: https://mchatscreen.com/. Accessed October 20, 2021.

[47] Massachusetts General Hospital. Pediatric symptom checklist. Available at: https://www.massgeneral.org/psychiatry/treatments-and-services/pediatric-symptom-checklist. Accessed October 20, 2021.

[48] Health Resources & Services Administration. PHQ-9: modified for teens. Available at: https://www.hrsa.gov/behavioral-health/phq-9-modified-teens. Accessed October 20, 2021.

[49] The Columbia Lighthouse Project. Screener with triage for primary care. Available at: https://cssrs.columbia.edu/documents/c-ssrs-screener-triage-primary-care/. Accessed October 21, 2021.

[50] University of Pittsburgh, Department of Psychiatry. Assessment instruments. Available at: https://www.pediatricbipolar.pitt.edu/resources/instruments. Accessed October 20, 2021.

[51] Kaye DL, Fornarib V, Scharf M. Description of a multi-university education and collaborative care child psychiatry access program: New York State's CAP PC. Gen Hosp Psychiatry 2017;48:32–6.

[52] Wissow LS, Nvan G, Chandna J, et al. Integrating children's mental health into primary care. Johns Hopkins University; 2016. Available at: https://jhu.pure.elsevier.com/en/publications/integrating-childrens-mental-health-into-primary-care. Accessed September 28, 2021.

[53] Learn about the collaborative care model. Available at: https://www.psychiatry.org/psychiatrists/practice/professional-interests/integrated-care/learn. Accessed October 21, 2021.

[54] National Network of Child Psychiatry Programs. Our story. Available at: https://www.nncpap.org/about-us. Accessed October 21, 2021.

[55] Behavioral health integration in physician practices. Available at: https://www.ama-assn.org/delivering-care/public-health/behavioral-health-integration-physician-practices. Accessed October 21, 2021.

[56] Tyler ET, Hulkover RL, Kaminski JW. Behavioral health integration in pediatric primary care: considerations and opportunities for policymakers, planners, and providers. New York, NY: Millbank Memorial Fund; 2017. Available at: https://www.milbank.org/publications/behavioral-health-integration-in-pediatric-primary-care-considerations-and-opportunities-for-policymakers-planners-and-providers/.

[57] Yonek J, Lee CM, Harrison A, et al. Key components of effective pediatric integrated mental health care models. JAMA Pediatr 2020;174(5):487; https://doi.org/10.1001/jamapediatrics.2020.0023.

[58] Petts R, Shahidullah JD, Kettlewell PW, et al. As a pediatrician, i don't know the second, third, or fourth thing to do: a qualitative study of pediatric residents' training and experiences in behavioral health. Int J Health Sci Educ 2018;12(1). Available at: https://dc.etsu.edu/cgi/viewcontent.cgi?article=1075&context=ijhse. Accessed September 28, 2021.

[59] McKague DK, Beebe SL, McNelis AM, et al. Lack of pediatric mental health clinical experiences among fnp students. Arch Psychiatr Nurs 2021;35(3):267–70; https://doi.org/10.1016/j.apnu.2021.03.008.

[60] Triple P. positive parenting programs. Available at: https://www.triplep.net/glo-en/home/. Accessed October 20, 2021.

[61] The incredible years. Available at: https://incredibleyears.com/. Accessed October 21, 2021.

[62] Totsika V, Mandair S, Lindsay G. Comparing the effectiveness of evidence-based parenting programs on families of children with and without special educational needs: short-term and long-term gains. Front Educ 2017; https://doi.org/10.3389/feduc.2017.00007.

[63] CEBC Overview. The California evidence-based clearinghouse for child welfare information and resources for child welfare professionals. Available at: https://www.cebc4c-w.org/leadership/overview/. Accessed October 21, 2021.

[64] NAMI OnDemand Class for Parents and Grandparents Self-Paced Start Anytime. National alliance on mental illness. Available at: https://nami-delaware-and-morrow-counties.events.idloom.com/basicsondemand. Accessed October 21, 2021.

[65] Brister T, Cavaleri S, Olin SS, et al. An evaluation of the NAMI Basics Program. J Child Fam Stud 2012;(21):439–42; https://doi.org/10.1007/s10826-011-9496-6.

[66] Anxiety Canada. My Anxiety Plan (MAP) for children and teens. Available at: https://maps.anxietycanada.com/en/courses/child-map/. Accessed October 22, 2021.

[67] Creating Opportunities for Personal Empowerment (COPE). Evidence-based programs for primary and secondary schools, universities, primary care practices, healthcare systems and professionals, parents and children. Available at: https://www.cope2thrive.com/. Accessed October 22, 2021.

[68] American Psychiatric Association. App advisor evaluation model. Available at: https://www.psychiatry.org/psychiatrists/practice/mental-health-apps/the-app-evaluation-model. Accessed October 21, 2021.

[69] Stoyanov SR, Hides L, Kavanagh DJ, et al. Mobile app rating scale: a new tool for assessing the quality of health mobile apps. JMIR mHealth uHealth 2015;3(1). https://mhealth.jmir.org/.

[70] Licholai GP, Feuerstein S MD, JD. The expanding role of digital therapeutics in mental health. The Psychiatric Times; 2021. Available at: https://www.psychiatrictimes.com/view/the-expanding-role-of-digital-therapeutics-in-mental-health. Accessed October 20, 2021.

[71] Baez D. Cognitive behavioural therapy app reduces symptoms of depression in adolescents NTK Institute. NTK Institute; 2021. Available at: https://ntk-institute.org/article/cognitive-behavioural-therapy-app-reduces-symptoms-of-depression-in-adolescents. Accessed October 18, 2021.

[72] The Reach Institute. The resource for advancing children's mental health. Available at: https://www.thereachinstitute.org/. Accessed October 21, 2021.

[73] The Ohio State College of Nursing. KySS mental health fellowship: child and adolescent (Online). Available at: https://nursing.osu.edu/offices-and-initiatives/office-continuing-education/kyss-mental-health-fellowship-child-and. Accessed October 21, 2021.

[74] U.S. Department of Health and Human Services. Mental health: a report of the surgeon general. Rockville, MD: U.S. Department of Health and Human Services, Substance Abuse and Mental Health Services Administration, Center for Mental Health Services, National Institutes of Health, National Institute of Mental Health; 1999.

Grief in Children

Meghan Tracewski, MSN, RN, CPNP, ACHPN[a],*,
Katie Scarlett, CCLS[b]

[a]Pediatric Advanced Care Team, Children's Healthcare of Atlanta, 1405 Clifton Road NE, Atlanta, GA 30322, USA; [b]Child Life, Children's Healthcare of Atlanta, 1001 Johnson Ferry Road NE, Atlanta, GA 30342, USA

Keywords

- Loss • Bereavement in childhood • Death concepts • Healthy grief
- Family functioning

Key points

- Children experience grief in relation to their developmental understanding of loss and the finality of death.
- The family unit is integral in promoting a nurturing environment that facilitates open conversation to process the complex emotions surrounding death.
- The primary care provider is an important resource for guiding the child and family through the evolution of grief and bereavement.
- Primary care providers and caregivers need to be prepared to lead discussions about death with children.
- This article offers a framework for applying knowledge of the pediatric grief experience to interventions that promote healthy responses to loss.

CLINICAL VIGNETTE

Mrs Lu is a 47-year-old patient in today for her annual examination. In gathering her social history, she reveals her father was diagnosed with stage IV pancreatic cancer two months ago and enrolled in hospice services last week. She is unsure how to tell her children ages 4, 8, and 14 years. They know that "Grandpa is sick," but not the extent. She is especially concerned about her 8-year-old given his close connection to Grandpa. Mrs Lu asks for your advice about what to tell the children and how to include them in the final stage of his life (Box 1 and 2).

*Corresponding author. E-mail address: Meghan.Tracewski@choa.org

https://doi.org/10.1016/j.yfpn.2021.12.012

You advise Mrs Lu each of her children will have a unique experience of Grandpa's death. They may have different questions and need to be involved in their own ways. Encourage her to talk to them together while devoting time for separate conversations. She should explore a legacy project they can complete with Grandpa or consider visiting him to say goodbye.

You ask Mrs Lu if she has thought about the children attending the memorial service following Grandpa's death. She is unsure what the "right" thing to do is. You suggest she ask each child if they want to attend and assign a trusted family member or friend to them. She should provide anticipatory guidance about what they may see at the funeral including his body, people crying as well as reassurance that this is normal, and it is okay to be sad.

INTRODUCTION

Death is not the opposite of life but an innate part of life.

—Haruki Murakami [1].

Death is part of the life cycle that will impact all children to varying degrees. It is estimated that 5% to 7% of the pediatric population will experience the death of a close family member before the age of 18 [2,3]. How a child experiences death and loss can be affected by their relationship to the deceased, how their family unit copes with loss, and the circumstances surrounding the death [4–7]. Other major factors that influence the child's grief include their understanding of the irreversibility of death [8] and how they are guided through the grieving process [9].

Clinicians and caregivers report feeling uncomfortable or ill-equipped at initiating discussions with children about difficult topics such as death [10]. Many adults feel it is their responsibility to shield children from sadness [9,11,12]. Some erroneously believe a child is incapable of understanding loss and therefore should not be included in adult conversations [11]. Others avoid talking about death because they do not know how to approach these discussions or fear being asked questions they may not possess the answers to [8,10,12]. The consequences of isolating a child from conversations about death can be grief that does not evolve [12–14] or dissolution of trust between caregivers and the child [4,8]. Avoiding the acknowledgment of a child's grief experience denies them the ability to establish a future in which they can live a healthy new normal without the deceased in it [15].

The primary care clinician has a vital role in providing developmentally appropriate anticipatory guidance to families faced with death [4]. In collaboration with the caregiver, the provider can help to create a space where a child is given permission to name, address, and process the complex emotions of loss. In following the lead of the child, the caregiver can most effectively address their needs [12]. Research has shown the more open caregivers are at having conversations with their children the less shame a child has for feeling what they do [14,16]. When included in a healthy, supportive shared bereavement journey with their family [4] the child is given the ability to adapt, recover, and heal from loss [15,17].

The provider should have comfort in initiating conversations with children, validating normal grief reactions, and identifying situations that precipitate impaired grief experiences [9]. The primary care clinician must also be a resource to families throughout the evolving grief process. They can use their knowledge of childhood development to lead discussions in a developmentally appropriate manner. They can use their relationship with the family to develop a deeper understanding of how everyone is coping with loss. Together the clinician, the caregiver, and child can successfully navigate this journey.

This article reviews theories of grief and the process of acclimating to life without the deceased as it pertains to a child's developmental conceptualization and comprehension of death. This article offers a framework for assessing family coping to best support the grieving child and tools to improve provider comfort in navigating difficult discussions with the pediatric patient. We will review ways to engage in the conversation and offer resources to help continue to support the entire family.

OVERVIEW OF GRIEF

Grief is defined as one's emotional response to bereavement, the loss or death of something or someone [8,18–20]. It has no definite trajectory nor predictable duration. It is a continual evolution as the bereaved individual adjusts to a life without the deceased in it. Early research in the field of death and bereavement defined concrete, linear states one must work through [21,22]. As more research is conducted on grief, it is felt to be a more dynamic process in which the individual ebbs and flows through the complex emotions over time [23,24] (Table 1). For a person to evolve in grief, one must move through tasks that bring about a transformation in one's self and their relationship to the world [5,6,14,25]. There are times during which the individual's growth is related to resolving the past and others where it is focused on recovering for the future [20]. For a child, this process can take years and happens in the context of their family unit [12].

The consistent theme across grief theories is the individual's ability to process the loss of the deceased in their life. For children, they must first understand the concept of death before they can begin their own grief journey. This must involve a recognition everyone dies, death is irreversible, one ceases to function after death (ie, the opposite of life), and something extraneous to their thoughts and behavior caused the death [9,10]. This work is facilitated by introducing the concept of death before it impacts the child's day to day and what it means to be alive through conversations or reading books on the subject [26]. Prepare the child by teaching them about the life cycle of living things in their everyday environment, such as plants and animals [26,27].

If you are approached with questions on helping a child with death, it would be important to assess how the caregiver(s) and family are coping. A study on the interconnectedness of a surviving caregiver and child

Table 1 Theories and tasks of grief	
Theory	**Stages or tasks**
Bowlby Phase Model (1980) [21]	Shock
	Searching
	Despair
	Recovery
The Five Stages of Grief (1969) [22]	Denial
	Anger
	Depression
	Bargaining
	Acceptance
Tasks of Mourning (1982) [14]	Accepting the loss is real
	Feeling the pain of loss
	Adjustment to life without the deceased
	Shifting energy from the deceased to other relationships
Multidimensional Grief Theory (2017) [25]	Separation Distress
	Existential/Identity Distress
	Circumstantial Distress
Dual Process Model of Coping (1999) [20]	Loss Oriented Coping (negative and positive)
	Recovery Oriented Coping (negative and positive)

describes grief after death as a shared journey. How well the surviving caregiver coped with the death influenced the child's grief [5,9,13]. If the caregivers tasked with supporting the child through a death have challenged coping themselves, then the downstream permeation or effect can have lasting implications on the child. The child must be allowed to grieve alongside their loved ones and not be shielded from it. The caregiver with a strong support network will have more emotional availability to help their child [13]. When providing guidance on supporting a child through grief, it would be important to assess the family structure and how they in general are coping with the loss (Box 1).

Encourage the caregiver to reflect on the first time they remember experiencing death of a loved one. Fitzgerald calls this to be taking a "death history," in which the caregiver reminds themselves how they felt, what helped them, what did not help, and what information was shared with them during their childhood exposure to death [26]. This process can help the caregiver to approach their child by using their own experiences and the recognition they, too, got through death.

As the provider, you may be looked to as the expert in initiating difficult discussions about the finality of death or answering questions about what a child should and should not be allowed to do. Death may lead to changes in routine, especially if the death is in a parent or primary care giver. Participation in purposeful rituals has been shown to provide individuals with a meaningful way to regain control during a time that feels chaotic [4,17]. Many experts agree that children as young as preschool age should be

Box 1: Suggested questions for the caregiver

- Who would you define to be in your family unit? Extended family?
- What is [the child's] relationship to the deceased?
- What discussions have you had with your child about death previously?
- How will death impact [the child's] functional life? Will you have to relocate or find another job?
- How has death impacted you?
- What is your first memory of death? What went well? What did not?
- Who is available to support you?
- Who, beside yourself, is available to support [the child] in the family or community?
- Has your family dealt with death in the past?
- How has your family dealt with difficult things, including death, before?
- What role does your culture or religion play in the rituals surrounding death?

Data from Refs [8,9,11,27]

prepared for and provided with the choice to participate in any rituals surrounding the death of a loved one [28–31]. Similar to other rituals, such as weddings or graduations, end-of-life rituals are important occasions to provide opportunity for family support. End-of-life rituals can also aid in the confirmation of the finality of death [32]. How to navigate this requires a foundational understanding of how a child processes death and works through their grief from a developmental perspective. Keep in mind that this is a guideline and not an absolute as mastery of developmental skills and comprehension of death is unique to the child [10].

In breaking any type of bad news or engaging in a difficult conversation, you first need to take a deep breath. This conversation is not easy for the child to have, either. Explaining death to a child is a complex task, for even the skilled clinician [8]. As with any difficult discussion, the words may not be perfect. The words you choose cannot make the information easier or the situation better. A child may not remember what was said, yet they will remember how they felt [31]. The situation is made better with a trusted, approachable presence. Be gentle and allow the child's pace and inquisition to lead the flow of the conversation [26]. Start the discussion by having them tell you what they know, what they are thinking about, and what may be worrying them the most [10,26].

CONCEPTUALIZATION OF GRIEF ACROSS THE PEDIATRIC AGE SPECTRUM (TABLE 2)

Infant: Ages 0 to 1

Infants depend on their caregivers to respond to their cues and meet their basic needs at this stage in their development. The establishment of this

Table 2
Developmental theoretic framework

Age	Psychosocial development [33]		Cognitive development [34]		Death concept [27]
	Crisis	Outcomes	Stages	Outcomes	
0 1	Trust vs mistrust	Build trust with caregivers who provide consistent care. Absence can lead to mistrust.	Sensorimotor	Discover world through sensory exploration and motor movements. Object permanence through attachment bonds.	Aware of changes to environment and inconsistently met needs owing to death of or separation (physical/emotional) from primary caregiver.
2 3	Autonomy vs shame and doubt	Develop independence and seek physical control. Absence can lead to feelings of shame and doubt.	Preoperational	Understand world through egocentric symbolic play and magical thinking, characterized by centration, animism, and inability to recognize cause/effect.	Believe death is reversible and magical thinking may lead to denial. Inability to understand cause and effect combined with egocentrism may lead fear they were reason individual died.
4 5	Initiative vs guilt	Assert control in environment to develop sense of purpose. Absence or disapproval can lead to guilt.			May not have language to verbalize awareness of change in emotions around them or in self. Slight grasp of death as irreversible and part of the life cycle. Continued inability to understand concrete concepts leads to altered perception of reality.

Age	Psychosocial stage	Psychosocial development [33]		Cognitive development [34]
			Concrete operational	
6 7	Industry vs inferiority	Develop mastery of social and academic experiences. Absence or feelings of failure can lead to inferiority.	Uses concrete and logical thought perform operations and solve problems. Possess ability to differentiate between animate and inanimate objects. As egocentrism lessens the ability to develop peer relationships strengthens.	Death is a real concept that may be personified as a ghost or monster rather than a state of being. Death happens because of something and can be avoided at times.
8 9 10 11 12				
13 14 15 16 17 18	Identity vs role confusion	Develop sense of self. Absence can lead to role confusion and decreased sense of self.	Formal operational Grasps abstract concepts. Able to integrate self into social constructs.	Death is understood to be absolute.

Adapted from Lanzel A, Brock KE. Children's views on death and dying: an overview and ethical focus on advance care planning communication with children. Journal of Pediatric Ethics. 2020;1(3):101-112. Available at http://ijpedethics.com/JPE%201-3.pdf; with permission.

trusting relationship is crucial to infants' social and emotional development [33,34]. Although the infant cannot understand death, they are aware of absences in or changes to their environment when their cues are not responded to and their needs remain unmet. This can happen when the infant is affected by the death of a primary caregiver or the death of someone beloved by the caregiver. An infant will notice if their primary caregiver is gone. They will also sense if their caregiver is suddenly emotional or distracted after experiencing a loss of their own [35]. A caregiver who themselves has unresolved grief will struggle to support their child [12]. The departure from what has been normal for the infant can be equated to a grief experience [21].

Manifestation of grief
Infants may show signs of distress through increased crying and fussiness. They tend to demonstrate amplified attachment to the primary or surviving caregiver and have difficulty coping with separation or strangers [31]. They may also exhibit changes in their eating and sleeping routines [9].

Recommendations for the caregiver
- Provide physical contact by holding and/or rocking infant
- Use eye contact to enhance sense of security and trust
- Create a soothing environment by singing or reading
- Maintain routines and allow for flexibility
- Include consistent, familiar caregivers
- Consider designating a surrogate caregiver during participation in end of life rituals that may distress the primary caregiver [14,32,35,36].

Toddler: Ages 1 to 3
The toddler has mastered sensorimotor development and established trust with their primary caregivers. As they progress into the preoperational stage of development the toddler is seeking independence [33] and uses symbolic play to express themselves [34]. They may have developed some words or short phrases; however, they lack the verbal skills to express their own emotions or respond to the emotions of others [37]. Toddlers cannot differentiate between the permanence of death and temporary separation [38].

Manifestation of grief
A toddler may show signs of distress similar to that of infants by regressing in their development. They may exhibit changes in their eating and sleeping routines as well as in their bowel and bladder habits [39]. Toddlers may display increased crying, biting, throwing, and separation and stranger anxiety [35]. Their experiences of grief tend to be sporadic and in small increments [40]. Toddlers may display these signs 1 minute, and then be happy or playful the next.

Recommendations for the caregiver
- The same interventions as with an infant to enhance trust and connection
- Avoid euphemisms such as lost, passed, or gone to sleep

- Use concrete words such as died, death, and dying
- Explain death in physiologic terms: absence of breathing, eating, playing, sleeping
- Anticipate repeated questioning by toddlers old enough to express themselves [31,32,35,36].

Preschool age child: Ages 3 to 5

Preschoolers continue to use symbolic thinking; they are unable to understand concrete logic and the perspective of others [34]. Children in this stage are egocentric and concerned about their own well-being or how events impact them [33]. They may wonder who will care for them when someone close to them dies. Their propensity for magical thinking may precipitate the belief they caused someone's death through their thoughts, words, or actions [34]. Similarly, they possess the power to bring a loved one back if they do good things [9,38]. Without concrete logic and with the presence of magical thinking, preschoolers may view death as reversible and have difficulty distinguishing it from sleep [38]. The older preschooler will start to develop the sense that death is irreversible. They may also imagine the funeral and other after death rituals to be worse than reality if not given the opportunity to participate or at least discuss [9].

Manifestation of grief

Play is central to the understanding and processing of death at this age. Preschoolers are learning emotional identification and may struggle to articulate what they feel [34]. This process may manifest as continued questioning about all aspects of death [26]. They may have more comfort in expressing thoughts and fears through play. For example, if a caregiver died in a motor vehicle accident, the preschooler may reenact their understanding of the situation with toy cars. Grieving preschoolers may regress in their development or exhibit changes in their routines or elimination habits. They may also display irritability, anger, aggression, or withdrawal from other people [39].

Recommendations for the caregiver

- Use concrete language to factually explain death
  - Grandpa died because his pancreas was sick. Your pancreas is a part of the inside of your body that helps to break down the food you eat to give your body energy.
- Clarify the child's wellness
  - Your pancreas is healthy. You cannot catch what Grandpa had.
- Diffuse magical thoughts
  - Nothing that you thought, said, or did caused Grandpa to die
- Expect repeated questions and provide honest answers
- Name and acknowledge the feelings of the child and caregivers
- Reinforce that it is okay to cry. It is a natural response to being sad
- Provide opportunities for emotional expression through conversation, play, and art
- Read books to promote emotional identification, processing, and understanding of death

- Consider designating a surrogate caregiver during participation in end-of-life rituals that may be distressing to the primary caregiver
- If a child does not want to attend a funeral, explore why, and clarify any false narratives they may have conjured in their magical thinking. Their rationale may not be what we think it is [32,35,36].

School age child: Ages 6 to 12

Peer relationships become increasingly important during the school age years [33]. Children experience decreased egocentrism and begin developing the ability to understand concrete logic, cause and effect, and that people experience other perspectives [34]. They may fear their own death and the death of loved ones as they start to view death as final and irreversible [38]. The school age child could have questions about religious or spiritual beliefs after death [41] or they may personify death by identifying it as a ghost or the Grimm Reaper [26,38].

Manifestation of grief
School-agers who have experienced a death close to them may show signs of distress by fearing their own death or the death of loved ones [35]. They may regress in their development [39] and display behaviors that they have not in a long time, or they may attempt to take on additional responsibilities or the behaviors of the deceased [35]. They may experience somatic symptoms, such as abdominal pain, headache, or fatigue [39]. Their inability to fully possess an understanding of death may manifest in continued questions. Grief may also manifest in school attendance or performance [9,26,39].

Recommendations for the caregiver
- The same interventions as with a preschool child to explain death, but provide more information as developmentally appropriate
- Ask open-ended questions to assess the child's thoughts and feelings
- Allow for religious and spiritual development
- Encourage the child to choose how to be involved in memorials and rituals at the time of death and on important anniversaries
- Provide opportunities for expression of feelings
- Inform your child's teacher about the death so they may monitor any changes in performance, engagement, or need for support while at school
- Explore peer support [26,32,35,38].

Adolescent: Ages 13 to 18

Adolescents are establishing a sense of self and identity in relation to their personal values, beliefs, and goals [33]. As they master abstract reasoning, they can conceptualize death to be permanent and inevitable [34,38]. Their attitude toward death may differ from their caregivers and they may struggle wanting to be both dependent on and independent from their family [4,24].

Manifestation of grief
Adolescents can display behaviors that vacillate between adult-like and child-like despite possessing a mature understanding of death. They may feel the

responsibility to assume adult roles and tasks then contrarily display isolating, self-centered, or risk-taking behaviors [25,35]. Because self-esteem is increasingly important during adolescence [33], the grieving teen may be self-conscious about being different from their peers because of their experiences with loss. They may not want to share their feelings to avoid being different than or to protect their caregivers from additional stressors and responsibilities [35].

Recommendations for the caregiver
- Include the adolescent in conversations related to death
- Provide opportunities to ask questions and share feelings or concerns
- Clarify roles and let your adolescent know that they are not expected to assume adult responsibilities if not appropriate
- Encourage support from peers or other adults, including mental health professionals
- Recommend creative outlets for expression of feelings
- Validate feelings [32,35,36].

Assessing for concerning grief behaviors

As mentioned elsewhere in this article, grief has no exact trajectory or timeline. One does not get over this loss. One heals from loss as they acclimate to life without the deceased. The provider and caregiver will need to monitor a grieving child to ensure they continue to exhibit healthy coping over time. They must also assess for situations that could precipitate a complicated grief experience such as mass casualty or traumatic death, the child's presence at death, and death related to the pandemic [9,10,12,42,43]. Possible signs a child is struggling with loss are as follows:

- Refusal to discuss anything related to the death
- Avoidance in using the deceased individual's name
- Creating a fantasy where the deceased never existed or is replaced by an imaginary friend
- Escalating destructive or reckless behaviors
- Lack of interest in activities that previously brought joy
- Unusual attempts to please others and avoid making them angry

Persistence in any of these behaviors would warrant referral to a mental health specialist. Any suspicion of suicidal ideation, concern for harm of others, or perseveration on one's own death would warrant emergent referral [9,26,42].

Much is still left to be learned about the long-term implications on grief and bereavement from the COVID-19 pandemic. There is evolving concern for the impending public mental health crisis it will cause for years to come. One can assume there will be complex grief reactions secondary to the sheer number of individuals affected as well as the complicated circumstances surrounding death and the post mortem experience of survivors. Unfortunately, many things known to promote healthy grief are not possible during the pandemic including saying goodbye to loved ones in the hospital, participation in rituals with others, attending funerals, and things as simple as a hug [43,44]. We would encourage you to remain up to date with local, state and national recommendations to provide guidance to the families you are working with.

SUMMARY

Death is a complex experience for an individual of any age. It comes with a range of emotions. A child's grief exists within the context of their family unit. Children's concept of death is continually evolving alongside their cognitive and psychosocial development.

Working with children and families during end of life experiences can be a challenging and emotional role for any healthcare professional. As you enter the conversations with caregivers and children be prepared to listen and receive questions knowing you may not be able to answer them all. A child may ask several why and how questions. Use your judgment about where the child's maturity and developmental level are to answer. It will help them to feel validated in their sadness; children who shielded from grief may feel their emotions should be hidden from others. The provision of family-centered care amid grief is a difficult and necessary role. With appropriate education and a comfort level in leading difficult conversations, the primary care provider can offer pivotal guidance and support to families and children. Grief does not have to be scary or unknown. It is not the provider's responsibility to fix the situation yet rather to allow a space where the child and the caregiver feel safe in their continuum of individual and collective experience of grief.

Disclosure

Nothing to disclose.

SUPPLEMENTARY DATA

Supplementary data related to this article can be found online at https://doi.org/10.1016/j.yfpn.2021.12.012.

References

[1] Murakami H. Norwegian Wood. New York: Vintage Books; 1987.

[2] Judi's house for grieving children and families. Available at: https://judishouse.org/. Accessed August 31, 2021.

[3] Palmer M, Saviet M, Tourish J. Understanding and supporting grieving adolescents and young adults. Pediatr Nurs 2016;42(6):275–81.

[4] Andriessen K, Mowll J, Lobb E, et al. Don't bother about me. The grief and mental health of bereaved adolescents. Death Stud 2018;42(10):607–15.

[5] Hill RM, Oosterhoff B, Layne CM, et al. Multidimensional grief therapy: pilot open trial of a novel intervention for bereaved children and adolescents. J Child Fam Stud 2019;28:3062–74.

[6] Kaplow JB, Layne CM, Saltzman WR, et al. Using multidimensional grief therapy to explore effects of deployment, reintegration, and death on military youth and families. Clin Child Fam Psychol Rev 2013;16(3):322–40.

[7] Kentor RA, Kaplow JB. Supporting children and adolescents following parental bereavement; guidance for healthcare professionals. Lancet Child Adolesc Health 2020;4:889–98.

[8] Riely M. Facilitating children's grief. J Sch Nurs 2003;19(4):212–8.

[9] Schonfeld DJ, Demaria T. Committee on psychosocial aspects of child and family health, disaster preparedness advisory council. Supporting the grieving child and family. Pediatrics 2016;138(3):e20162147; https://doi.org/10.1542/peds.2016-2147.

[10] Corr CA. Children's understandings of death, striving to understand death. In: Doka KJ, editor. Children mourning, mourning children. Hospice Foundation of America; 1995. p. 3–16.

[11] Contro N, Kreicbergs U, Reichard WJ, et al. Anticipatory grief and bereavement. In: Wolfe J, Hinds PS, Sourkes BM, editors. Textbook of interdisciplinary pediatric palliative care. Elsevier Saunders; 2011. p. 41–54.

[12] Doka KJ, editor. Living with grief: children, adolescents, and loss. Brunner/Mazel; 2000.

[13] Cipriano DJ, Cipriano MR. Factors underlying the relationship between parent and child grief. J Death Dying 2019;89(1):120–36.

[14] Worden J. Grief counselling and grief therapy: a handbook for the mental health practitioner. 5th. New York: Springer; 2018.

[15] Knight SJ, Emanuel LL. Loss, bereavement, and adaptation. In: Emanuel LL, Librach SL, editors. Palliative care core skills and clinical competencies. 2nd edition. St. Louis: Elsevier Saunders; 2011. p. 243–54.

[16] Lytje M, Dyregrov M. The price of loss: a literature review of the psychosocial and health consequences of childhood bereavement. Bereavement Care 2019;38(1):13–22.

[17] Norton MI, Gino F. Rituals alleviate grieving for loved ones, lovers, and lotteries. J Exp Psychol Gen 2014;143(1):266–72; https://doi.org/10.1037/a0031772.

[18] Miriam Webster dictionary. Available at: https://www.merriam-webster.com/. Accessed August 31, 2021.

[19] Balk D. Adolescent development and bereavement: an introduction. Prev Res 2011;18(3):3–10.

[20] Stroebe M, Schut H. The dual process model of coping with bereavement: rationale and description. Death Stud 1999;23(3):197–224.

[21] Bowlby J. Attachment and loss. 2nd edition. New York: Basic Books; 1982.

[22] Kübler-Ross E. On death and dying. New York: Scribner; 1969.

[23] Geronazzo-Alman L, Fan B, Duarte CS, et al. The distinctiveness of grief, depression, and posttraumatic stress: lessons from children after 9/11. J Am Acad Child Adolesc Psychiatry 2019;58(10):971–82.

[24] Mosher PJ. Everywhere and nowhere: grief in child and adolescent psychiatry and pediatric clinical populations. Child Adolesc Psychiatr Clin N Am 2018;27:109–24.

[25] Layne CM, Kaplow JB, Oosterhoff B, et al. The interplay between posttraumatic stress and grief reactions in traumatically bereaved adolescents: when trauma, bereavement, and adolescents converge. Adolesc Psychiatry 2017;7:220–39.

[26] Fitzgerald H. The grieving child. New York: Fireside; 1992.

[27] Lanzel A, Brock KE. Children's views on death and dying: an overview and ethical focus on advance care planning communication with children. J Pediatr Ethics 2020;1(3):101–12.

[28] Anderson B. Do children belong at funerals?. In: Adams DW, Deveau EJ, editors. Beyond the innocence of children: factors influencing children and adolescents/perceptions and attitudes toward death. New York: Routledge; 1995. p. 163–77.

[29] Grollman E. Explaining death to young children: some questions and answers. In: Grollman E, editor. Bereaved children and adolescents: a support guide for parents and professionals. Boston: Beacon Press; 1995. p. 3–19.

[30] Rando T. Grief, dying and death: clinical interventions for caregivers. Champaign: Research Press Company; 1984.

[31] Wolfet A. Helping children cope with grief. New York: Routledge; 1983.

[32] Thompson RH. The handbook of child life: a guide for pediatric psychosocial care. Springfield: Charles C Thomas; 2009.

[33] Erikson E. Children and society. New York: Norton; 1963.

[34] Piaget J. The theory of stages in cognitive development. Monterey: McGraw-Hill; 1969.

[35] Pearson L. Separation, loss, and bereavement. In: Broome M, Rollins J, editors. Core curriculum for the nursing care of children and their families. Pitman: Jannetti; 1999. p. 77–92.

[36] Rollins JA, Bolig R, Mahan CC. Meeting children's psychosocial needs across the healthcare continuum. Austin: PRO-ED, Inc; 2005.

[37] Hames CC. Helping infants and toddlers when a family member dies. J Hosp Palliat Nurs 2003;5:103–10.

[38] Speece MW, Brent SB. The acquisition of a mature understanding of three components of the concept of death. Death Stud 1992;16:211–29.

[39] The pediatrician and childhood bereavement. American Academy of Pediatrics. Committee on Psychosocial Aspects of Child and Family Health. Pediatrics 2000;105(2):445–7.

[40] Christ GH. Impact of development on children's mourning. Cancer Pract 2000;8:72–81.

[41] Shapiro ER. Grief as a family process: a developmental approach to clinical practice. New York: Guilford Press; 1994.

[42] Arizmendi BJ, O'Connor MF. What is normal in grief? Aust Crit Care 2014;28:58–62.

[43] Petry SE, Hughes D, Galanos A. Grief: the epidemic within an epidemic. Am J Hosp Palliat Med 2021;38(4):419–22.

[44] Centers for Disease Control. Guidance for COVID-19. 2021. Available at: https://www.cdc.gov/coronavirus/2019-ncov/communication/guidance.html. Accessed August 31, 2021.

Mind-Body Therapies for Children with Functional Abdominal Pain

Donna Marshall Moyer, PhD, RN, PCNS-BC[a],*,
Ann Sheehan, DNP, CPNP[b]

[a]Michigan State University, College of Nursing, Life Science Building, 1355 Bogue Street, A117C, East Lansing, MI 48824, USA; [b]Michigan State University, College of Nursing, Life Science Building, 1355 Bogue Street, A124, East Lansing, MI 48824, USA

Keywords
- Functional abdominal pain • Mind-body therapies • Complementary therapies
- Alternative therapies • Children

Key points
- There is growing evidence that mind-body therapies are effective in reducing pain and anxiety among children and adolescents with functional abdominal pain.
- Providers in family practice settings can recommend and implement several mind-body therapies in the care of children and adolescents with functional abdominal pain.
- Some mind-body therapies can be provided to children and families with minimal or no cost.
- Family practice providers should include mind-body therapies when developing the treatment plan of a child or adolescent diagnosed with functional abdominal pain.

INTRODUCTION

Providers in family practice will likely encounter children with chronic abdominal pain. The condition can be difficult to diagnose, and its management is frequently frustrating for the child, parent, and health care providers. In cases where no underlying pathology is identified, providers are left to manage a child's persistent pain without clear or complete direction, and a multimodal approach is required. This article provides an overview of functional

*Corresponding author. E-mail address: moyerd@msu.edu

https://doi.org/10.1016/j.yfpn.2021.12.013
2589-420X/22/© 2021 Elsevier Inc. All rights reserved.

abdominal pain (FAP) in children and describe several mind-body therapies that may be effective in treating those with the condition.

FUNCTIONAL ABDOMINAL PAIN
Diagnosis
Abdominal pain affects people of all ages and can be difficult to diagnose, as the differential diagnosis is quite large. Abdominal pain is typically characterized as acute or chronic. The acute form is often self-limiting and resolves within weeks. It is commonly related to infectious processes such as viral and bacterial gastroenteritis. In contrast, chronic abdominal pain persists for at least 2 months [1] and frequently includes a psychosocial component [2]. "Red flag" symptoms [3] that coincide with abdominal pain indicate the possibility of more serious pathology, and referral to a specialist should be considered in these cases (Box 1).

Abdominal pain accounts for roughly 10% of all emergency department visits, and a nonspecific diagnosis is made 41% of the time [4]. A diagnosis of FAP is applied when no organic cause is identified for the pain and symptoms cannot be attributed to another medical condition [5]. An organic cause of abdominal pain is identified in fewer than 10% of school-age children who seek medical care from a primary care provider [1]. Across all health care settings, 25% of children with complaints of abdominal pain are diagnosed with FAP [3]. The worldwide prevalence of FAP in children is 13.5% [6]. Girls and those with mental health conditions are disproportionately affected by FAP [6].

Box 1: Abdominal pain red flags

Persistent right upper quadrant pain

Persistent right lower quadrant pain

Pain that awakens the child from sleep

Dysphagia

Loss of appetite

Persistent vomiting

Arthralgia

Gastrointestinal bleeding

Nocturnal diarrhea

Involuntary weight loss

Deceleration of linear growth

Delayed puberty

Fever

Family history of irritable bowel syndrome, Celiac disease, or peptic ulcer disease

Data from Khan S. Functional abdominal pain in children. American College of Gastroenterology. August 2006. Updated December 2012. Accessed August 30, 2021. https://gi.org/topics/functional-abdominal-pain-in-children/.

FAP is one of many gut-brain interaction disorders in childhood [2]. It is identified by a cluster of symptoms, including abdominal pain experienced at least once per week for 2 or more months, pain that is episodic or continuous, pain that has an inconsistent pattern and location, and abdominal pain that is triggered from a variety of causes [1,3]. FAP is characterized as being "persistent or intermittent, waxing and waning or steady and unrelenting, sharp or dull, and worsened or unaffected by movement"[1][(p762)]. There are 4 main subtypes of FAP, including functional dyspepsia, irritable bowel disease, abdominal migraine, and FAP not otherwise specified. Those subtypes are characterized by a wide variety of symptoms (Box 2) that are not explained by any other diagnosis [7]. A normal physical examination is characteristic of FAP.

Contributing Factors

A biopsychosocial model of illness is used to describe the complex interrelationship of biological, psychological, and socioecological systems that contribute to

---

Box 2: Symptoms associated with functional abdominal pain disorders

Intermittent or continuous abdominal pain

Abdominal pain and cramping

Diffuse, moderate to severe abdominal pain that is midline and periumbilical

Pain unrelated to eating or other events

Bloating relieved with bowel movement

Change in appearance of bowel movement

Change in frequency of bowel movement

Mucus in bowel movement

Increased gas

Pain or burning in stomach after meals

Early satiety

Excessive burping

Nausea after meals

Pain in stomach relieved with meals

Headache

Anorexia

Nausea

Vomiting

Pallor

Data from Hyams JS, Di Lorenzo C, Saps M, Shulman RJ, Staiano A, van Tilburg M. Childhood functional gastrointestinal disorders: child/adolescent. *Gastroenterology,* 2016;150:1456-1468. doi:10.1053/j.gastro.2016.02.015.

the pain experience in FAP [2]. The enteric nervous system provides the biological mechanism for the pain that is experienced in FAP. The neural response can change with or without cause; however, abdominal infection, a traumatic life event, abdominal insult, or abuse can precipitate increased nerve sensitivity. Visceral hypersensitivity increases during times of high stress with a related increase in the child's perception of abdominal pain. Several psychosocial factors can also influence a child's pain experience and symptom expression in FAP, including family interactions and parent attention to gastrointestinal symptoms [2]. The interacting effects of the brain, gastrointestinal tract, and sociopsychological factors relate to the clinical expression of FAP [2]. The pathophysiology of FAP is therefore related to dysregulation of the brain-gut interaction and influenced by a host of social and psychological factors [1]. Simply put, children with FAP have an abnormal response to normal physiologic function, that is, pain is experienced or perceived with normal peristalsis.

Morbidity

FAP negatively affects a child's physical and psychological well-being and can adversely affect family functioning. Pain associated with FAP can be debilitating and for many children it interferes with school attendance, sports participation, and peer social interaction [3]. Distress caused by FAP may affect a child's emotional regulation, leading to depression or anxiety [3]. It is common for children with FAP to also experience pain in other areas of the body, further provoking anxiety, depression, and decreased health-related quality of life [8]. Family burden and frustration are prevalent for both parents and siblings of a child with FAP [9]. The child's parent can experience similar problems with emotional regulation due to feelings of helplessness. Consequently, the parent may also become anxious or depressed [10].

Treatment

The goal of FAP treatment of the child is pain reduction to a level that permits psychosocial health, full physical function, and improved quality of life. Given many contributing factors, treatment of children with FAP requires a multimodal approach. Medical treatments are based on the child's individual needs and should be selected in communication and collaboration with the patient and family. Education, reassurance, diet, medication, and psychological support are fundamental components of a treatment plan [2]. The child and parent should be taught that FAP is not life threatening and reassured that the child is in overall good physical health. It may be helpful for the patient and parent to know that 30% to 50% of FAP symptoms spontaneously resolve [1]. If the child's history warrants, a diet change may be helpful [3]. In some cases, pharmacologic treatment with antispasmodic medications, laxatives, or antacids may help with successful pain management [3]. An antidepressant may be necessary, if pain cannot otherwise be controlled [3]. Judicious use of medications is warranted, as there is little available evidence to support clinical decision-making [11].

Several nonpharmacologic strategies have been tried, including diet changes, prebiotics and probiotics, cognitive behavioral therapy, behavioral interventions, and alternative medicine [12]. Given the complex biopsychosocial cause of FAP, mind-body therapies may be effective at improving quality of life for young people with FAP and their families.

MIND-BODY THERAPIES
Overview
Complementary and integrative therapies are defined by the American Holistic Nurses' Association [13][(p114)] as, "A broad set of healthcare practices, therapies, and modalities that address the whole person—body, mind, emotion, spirit—rather than just signs and symptoms, which can replace or complement conventional nursing, biomedical, surgical, and pharmacologic treatments." Mind-body practices are a subset of complementary and integrative therapies that hold particular promise for pain management in children with FAP. Examples of mind-body practices include mindful meditation, guided imagery, hypnosis, yoga, tai chi, massage, prayer, art and music therapies, cognitive behavioral therapies, biofeedback, and relaxation techniques [13]. The overarching goal of mind-body therapies is to harness the power of thoughts, mental images, and attention to improve physical functioning and mental health [13].

Mind-Body Therapies in Children
The number of children in the United States who report using mind-body practices is growing. In analysis of data from the 2017 National Health Interview Survey (NHIS), Black and colleagues [14] (2018) found the percentage of children who used yoga and meditation increased significantly between 2012 and 2017. Children with chronic pain reportedly use mind-body therapies at an even higher rate [15,16]. Further analysis of the 2017 NHIS data revealed that children practiced meditation in several forms, including yoga, tai chi, qigong, mantra, mindfulness, and spiritual meditation [17].

Mind-body therapies have been investigated in treatment of several physiologic and psychological pediatric chronic conditions. For example, yoga has been used in asthma management [18], weight management [19], and treatment of anxiety and depression [20]. Mindfulness-based interventions have been used to treat symptom burden in children with cancer [21].

There is recent interest in the use of joint parent-child mind-body intervention delivery [22]. This approach makes intuitive sense in the case of FAP where family function is disrupted and there is parental frustration and anxiety related to the child's diagnosis [9].

Mind-Body Therapies for Functional Abdominal Pain
Several mind-body therapies have been studied in treatment of children with FAP, and a large percentage of children and families are already using them at home [23]. Hypnotherapy, cognitive behavioral theory, and biofeedback have been used by some providers with success, but specialized training is required, and out-of-pocket costs can be high for these therapies [24]. More accessible treatments include

mindful meditation, guided imagery, prayer, and yoga, as children and parents can be taught to use them at home by a knowledgeable and competent provider. A description of each of these therapies follows.

Mindful meditation is a technique that promotes attention and brings focus to the momentary present [25]. With the help of a guide, children focus on and accept their current thoughts, feelings, or sensations [26]. The goal of meditative practice is to increase control of mental processes in order to bring about calmness, physical relaxation, psychological balance, and overall health and well-being [27]. The American Academy of Pediatrics [28] recommends children and adolescents practice developmentally appropriate mindfulness or meditation activities daily. Sessions for preschool-age children may last only a few minutes, school-age children up to 10 minutes, whereas older children and adolescents can engage in the activity for up to 45 minutes at a time. Parents and siblings may also benefit from mindful meditation. By meditating together it is reasonable to expect there may be mutual calming, stress reduction, and improved family functioning, although little has been reported in the literature [22]. Knowledgeable providers can help children and parents learn skills of mindful meditation. There are books, reputable Web sites and mobile applications that can support meditative practice. Some free mobile applications that are a good source for guided meditations include Insight Timer; Smiling Mind; Mindfulness Daily; UCLA Mindful; and Stop, Breathe & Think.

Guided imagery is a mind-body technique that uses relaxation, breathing, and visualization to reduce stress and anxiety and improve overall well-being [29]. Imagery techniques can be especially effective with children, as a vivid imagination evokes elaborate mental imagery. General steps include getting into a relaxed and comfortable body position, using a focused breathing pattern, bringing the image to mind using all 5 senses, and spending time exploring the mental representation [29]. The goal is to use a mental image to bring about positive feelings that bring about physiologic change, so the imagery should involve a place or experience the child finds pleasing [29,30]. The recommended frequency of guided imagery therapy has not been established. However, the ability to bring to mind a clear mental representation requires practice, so short daily sessions may be warranted. Written scripts, audio recordings, and reputable Web sites provide families with resources to practice guided imagery at home.

Prayer is a form of spiritual healing in which children find strength, calmness, tranquility, and comfort [31]. Unlike other mind-body therapies, there is evidence that praying together promotes healthy family relationships [32]. When spirituality and faith practices are important to the child and family, prayer could play an important role in minimizing family dysfunction associated with a child's FAP. Parents may want to reach out to their chaplain or other religious leader for spiritual support [31].

Yoga is a series of body postures that are performed with a focus on the flow of breathing and internal reflection [33]. Tai chi and qigong are related forms of meditative movement that involve dynamic body movement in a more flowing sequence [34]. All forms of meditative movement seek to promote calmness, increase focus, and bring balance to the body, mind, and spirit. Children and parents can learn yoga from a certified instructor, but that results in out-of-pocket costs to the family. Books, online videos, or community outreach programs allow yoga practice free of charge [35].

For children with FAP, regular practice ensures that mind-body skills are developed and can then be used to manage acute pain episodes. All mind-body therapies require commitment and practice by the child and parents. Providers should discuss integrative therapy options, including any past experience, with children and families to identify the best method to include in the treatment plan. Several factors contribute to patients' decision to include mind-body or other integrative therapies into management of FAP, including provider influence, social influence, accessibility and insurance coverage, lifestyle, and philosophic or religious beliefs [23]. A consistent and trusted provider-patient relationship provides the therapeutic foundation for successful treatment of a child's FAP [2,36].

RECOMMENDATIONS FOR PRACTICE

Mind-body therapies are congruent with a holistic approach to care. Implementation of mind-body therapies requires knowledge, skill, and competence in their delivery. All providers who have been trained in academic degree programs or postlicensure programs and maintained competence in mind-body therapies can and should incorporate the interventions in the context of holistic nursing practice [13]. Providers are encouraged to become knowledgeable and competent in a variety of mind-body therapies, as one form has not been proven more effective than another and children respond differently.

Training and Safety

Providers have a duty to manage pain and suffering by applying individualized, evidence-based treatment modalities [37]. In order to individualize care, providers need to understand and maintain competence in a broad range of therapies. Many programs of nursing and medical education have incorporated integrative therapies, including mind-body interventions, into their curricula. However, most do not teach content that is specific to the pediatric population, and additional training may be needed [16]. Training, certification, and licensure requirements vary by state, and health care providers are cautioned to know the laws in their state and practice accordingly [38]. Comanagement of FAP with a certified or specially trained provider can be helpful for providers with limited training in integrative therapies and mind-body practices.

It has been demonstrated that children can and do practice multiple forms of mind-body therapies. The therapies are generally considered safe when implemented by knowledgeable providers [28,39]. However, integrative therapies are not without risk. Children with trauma history, for example, may experience increased anxiety or other forms of emotional distress in response to mindfulness and imagery [39]. Some individuals report feeling short of breath when they focus on breathing or deep diaphragmatic breathing [30]. There is also a lack of safety data reporting related to integrative therapies that is concerning [16,40]. Patients should be instructed to stop any treatment that is not achieving the desired effect. Providers should consider the risk versus benefit of each proposed therapy before their implementation and coordinate care with a mental health specialist when appropriate.

Access

Mind-body therapies can be used in a variety of health care settings and across the continuum of care. To improve access, in-person and virtual modes of intervention delivery are recommended options for relaxation and mindfulness interventions [41,42]. There are a wide variety of mobile health resources that can be used by children and families at home without cost. Careful vetting of mobile applications and online content before recommending them to a child and family is important, as some are of poor quality [26].

When making recommendation to include a mind-body practice in a child's plan of care, the child's age, developmental level, and interests should be considered. Family resources should also be taken into account. Depending on the specific therapy, costs are not often covered by insurance companies and can result in significant out-of-pocket expenses for families. A detailed discussion of coding and reimbursement is beyond the scope of this article but are a consideration for providers who recommend mind-body therapies. Although several payers do not reimburse for specialized holistic practitioners services, family practice providers can receive payment for education and counseling related to mind-body therapies in the course of a clinic visit.

Many therapies do not require frequent appointments or face-to-face interaction with a holistic health specialist. Providers who are knowledgeable of mind-body interventions can teach them to children and parents as a form of self-management that can be practiced and used at home. Once learned, the intervention is free of cost and always available to the child. Children and their parents can be taught multiple mind-body therapies, so a variety of options are available to manage pain events.

Case study

A case study illustrates how providers can incorporate mind-body therapies into the treatment plan of a child with FAP. Consider Cassie, a 12-year old girl being seen in the family practice clinic with a 4-month history of recurrent abdominal pain. Cassie experiences pain 3 to 4 days per week, with each pain event lasting between 30 minutes and several hours. She describes the pain as intermittent, with moderate to severe cramping across a large diffuse area of her middle and lower abdomen. On physical examination, she is of normal weight and height, and her physical assessment parameters are all within normal limits. She reports having a daily bowel movement, with occasional nausea or diarrhea during or following painful episodes. The abdominal pain does not seem to coincide with meals or other regular activity.

From a psychosocial perspective, Cassie is in sixth grade and reports having a best friend. Her parents are divorced and share physical custody of Cassie and her 14-year-old brother. Cassie lives with her mother during the school week and with her father on the weekends. She does well in school but finds some of her classes difficult. She has experienced the abdominal pain at school and reports having come home from school early on 3 days in the past month. Cassie's abdominal pain has started to interfere with participation on her soccer team. She has never experienced pain during soccer practice or a game. However, she states she is "scared she might" and skipped practice twice in the last 2 weeks.

Given abdominal pain absent any other physical findings, the provider makes a diagnosis of FAP. The condition is explained to Cassie and her mother, and they are provided reassurance that FAP is not life threatening and often self-limiting. The provider asks Cassie and her mother if they have tried any treatments at home. Cassie reports she usually lays down in her room and attempts to rest until the pain subsides. Her mother states that she started having Cassie take an over-the-counter probiotic each morning, which may have helped "a little."

The provider explains the relationship between stress and painful episodes in FAP and asks Cassie if she has ever used mindful meditation or other practices to reduce stress. Cassie reports that she "learned some things" in a school health class but has never used any of the strategies at home. Cassie and her mother state they are open to learning more about mindfulness and meditation.

The provider asks Cassie and her mother if they would like to try a brief meditative exercise. The provider dims the lights in the examination room and instructs them to sit comfortably with their backs straight, feet on the floor, and hands at their sides or on their laps. The provider prompts them to close their eyes and focus on their relaxed breathing. They complete the 4-minute guided meditation, *Simply Be* by Courtney Bohlman [43], from the Insight timer mobile application. After completing the meditation, the provider discusses their experience with the meditation. Cassie and her mother report feeling calm and think they will be able to use mindful meditation at home. The provider assesses the family's resources and determines that Cassie does not have a mobile phone with Internet access. However, her mother does have a phone and agrees to download a meditation application and join Cassie with daily practice. They are provided with a list of free mobile meditation applications.

In developing a treatment plan, the provider recommends Cassie continue taking the probiotic, because she feels like it may be helping. In addition to the probiotic, Cassie is encouraged to engage in regular activities of a healthy lifestyle, including adequate sleep, a balanced diet, and daily physical activity. She is encouraged to maintain her regular routine, including school and soccer related activities. Cassie's mother is encouraged to avoid frequent attention or focus on the abdominal pain. Finally, Cassie is encouraged to engage in some form of guided meditation for at least 10 minutes each day for the next 2 weeks and then return to the clinic for reevaluation of her FAP symptoms.

SUMMARY

FAP is a common condition of children and adolescents and is associated with several negative physical and psychological health outcomes. Because the diagnosis of FAP is based on symptomatology and no structural or physiologic cause is identified, it can be difficult to manage. There is growing evidence that mind-body therapies are a safe and effective way to manage FAP in children. Children and parents can use some mind-body therapies with little or no cost. A growing number of children are using mind-body therapies as a form of self-management of the condition. It is important for nurses in family practice to be knowledgeable so they can provide guidance on their use. Family practice providers should work with children diagnosed with FAP and their families to include mind-body therapies into a holistic treatment plan.

CLINICS CARE POINTS

- Children with functional abdominal pain benefit from multimodal intervention that includes mind-body therapies.
- Mindful meditation, guided imagery, prayer, and yoga are mind-body therapies can be adapted for use by children across the developmental spectrum.
- There may be benefit for families that participate in mind-body therapies with their children.

CONFLICT OF INTEREST

The authors declare they have no commercial or financial conflicts of interest associated with the content of this article. The authors have not received external financial support for the preparation or publication of this article.

References

[1] Gershman G. Abdominal pain. In: Berkowitz C, editor. Berkowitz's pediatrics: a primary care approach. 5th edition. American Academy of Pediatrics; 2014. p. 761–6.

[2] Drossman DA. Functional gastrointestinal disorders: history, pathophysiology, clinical features, and Rome IV. Gastroenterology 2016;150:1262–79.

[3] Khan S. Functional abdominal pain in children. Am Coll Gastroenterol 2006. Available at: https://gi.org/topics/functional-abdominal-pain-in-children/. Accessed August 30, 2021.

[4] Macaluso C, McNamara R. Evaluation and management of acute abdominal pain in the emergency department. Int J Gen Med 2012;5:789–97.

[5] McClellan N, Ahlawat R. Functional abdominal pain in children. StatPearls. 2021. Available at: https://www.ncbi.nlm.nih.gov/books/NBK537298/. Accessed August 30, 2021.

[6] Korterink J, Diederen K, Benninga M, et al. Epidemiology of pediatric functional abdominal pain disorders: a meta-analysis. PLOS ONE 2015;10(5):e0126982.

[7] Hyams JS, Di Lorenzo C, Saps M, et al. Childhood functional gastrointestinal disorders: child/adolescent. Gastroenterology 2016;150:1456–68.

[8] Chumpitazi BP, Palermo TM, Hollier JM, et al. Multisite pain is highly prevalent in children with functional abdominal pain disorders and is associated with increased morbidity. J Pediatr 2021; https://doi.org/10.1016/j.jpeds.2021.04.059.

[9] Brekke M, Brodwall A. Understanding parents' experiences of disease course and influencing factors: a 3-year follow-up qualitative study among parents of children with functional abdominal pain. BMJ Open 2020;10; https://doi.org/10.1136/bmjopen-2020-037288.

[10] Calvano C, Warschburger P. Quality of life among parents seeking treatment for their child's functional abdominal pain. Qual Life Res 2018;27(10):2557–70.

[11] Martin AE, Newlove-Delgado TV, Abbott RA, et al. Pharmacological interventions for recurrent abdominal pain in childhood. Cochrane Database Syst Rev 2017;3(3); https://doi.org/10.1002/14651858.CD010973.pub2.

[12] Rutten JM, Korterink JJ, Venmans LM, et al. Nonpharmacologic treatment of functional abdominal pain disorders: a systematic review. Pediatrics 2015;135(3):522–35.

[13] American Holistic Nurses' Association. Holistic nursing: scope and Standards of practice. 3rd edition. American Nurses Association; 2019.

[14] Black LI, Barnes PM, Clarke TC, et al. NCHS data brief, no 324: use of yoga, meditation, and Chiropractors among U.S. Children aged 4–17 years. National Center for Health Statistics; 2018.

[15] Groenewald CB, Beals-Erickson SE, Ralston-Wilson J, et al. Complementary and alternative medicine use by children with pain in the United States. Acad Pediatr 2017;17(7):785–93.

[16] McClafferty H, Vohra S, Bailey M, et al. Pediatric mind-body medicine. Pediatrics 2017;140(3); https://doi.org/10.1542/peds.2017-1961.

[17] Wang C, Li K, Gaylord S. Prevalence, patterns, and predictors of mediation use among U.S. children: results from the National Health Interview Survey. Complement Ther Med 2019;43:271–6.

[18] Lack S, Brown R, Kinser P. An integrative review of yoga and mindfulness-based approaches for children and adolescents with asthma. J Pediatr Nurs 2020;52:76–81.

[19] Dai CL, Sharma M, Chen CC, et al. Yoga as an alternative therapy for weight management in child and adolescent obesity: a systematic review and implications for research. Altern Ther Health Med 2021;27(1):48–55.

[20] James-Palmer A, Anderson EZ, Zucker L, et al. Yoga as an intervention for the reduction of symptoms of anxiety and depression in children and adolescents: a systematic review. Front Pediatr 2020;8:78.

[21] Tomlinson D, Sung L, Vettese E, et al. Mindfulness-based interventions for symptom management in children and adolescents with cancer: a systematic review. J Pediatr Oncol Nurs 2020;37(6):423–30.

[22] Guenther CH, Stephens RL, Ratliff ML, et al. Parent-child mindfulness-based training: a feasibility and acceptability study. J Evid Based Integr Med 2021;26:1–11.

[23] Ciciora SL, Yildiz VO, Jin WY, et al. Complementary and alternative medicine use in pediatric functional abdominal pain disorders at a large academic medical center. J Pediatr 2020;227:53–9.

[24] Gupta S, Schaffer G, Saps M. Pediatric irritable bowel syndrome and other functional abdominal pain disorders: An update of non-pharmacological treatment. Expert Rev Gastroenterol Hepatol 2018;12(5):447–56.

[25] Perry-Parrish C, Copeland-Linder N, Webb L, et al. Mindfulness-based approaches for children and youth. Curr Probl Pediatr Adolesc Health Care 2016;46:172–8.

[26] Gross CR, Christopher MS, Reilly-Spong M. Meditation. In: Lindquist R, Snyder M, Tracy MF, editors. Complementary & alternative therapies in nursing. 8th edition. Springer Publishing Company; 2018. p. 177–200.

[27] National Center for Complementary and Mind-body Health. Meditation: in depth. 2016. Available at: https://www.nccih.nih.gov/health/meditation-in-depth. Accessed August 30, 2021.

[28] American Academy of Pediatrics, Section on Integrative Medicine. Just breathe: the importance of meditation breaks for kids. 2017. Available at: https://www.healthychildren.org/

English/healthy-living/emotional-wellness/Pages/Just-Breathe-The-Importance-of-Meditation-Breaks-for-Kids.aspx. Accessed August 30, 2021.

[29] Krau S. The multiple uses of guided imagery. Nurs Clin North Am 2020;55:467–74.

[30] Fitzgerald M, Langevin M. Imagery. In: Lindquist R, Snyder M, Tracy MF, editors. Complementary & alternative therapies in nursing. 8th edition. Springer Publishing Company; 2018. p. 81–108.

[31] Rossato L, Ullán AM, Scorsolini-Comin F. Religious and spiritual practices used by children and adolescents to cope with cancer. J Relig Health 2021; https://doi.org/10.1007/s10943-021-01256-z.

[32] Chelladurai JM, Dollahite DC, Marks LD. "The family that prays together...": relational processes associated with regular family prayer. J Fam Psychol 2018;32(7):849–59.

[33] Stephens I. Medical yoga therapy. Children 2017;4(12); https://doi.org/10.3390/children4020012.

[34] Jahnke R, Larkey L, Rogers C, et al. A comprehensive review of health benefits of qigong and tai chi. Am J Health Promot 2010;24(6):e1–25.

[35] Cameron ME, Cheung CK. Yoga. In: Lindquist R, Snyder M, Tracy MF, editors. Complementary & alternative therapies in nursing. 8th edition. Springer Publishing Company; 2018. p. 151–61.

[36] Galdston MR, John RM. Mind over gut: psychosocial management of pediatric functional abdominal pain. J Pediatr Health Care 2016;30(6):535–45.

[37] ANA Ethics Advisory Board. ANA position statement: the ethical responsibility to manage pain and the suffering it causes. Online J Issues Nurs 2018;24(1); https://doi.org/10.3912/OJIN.Vol24No01PoSCol01.

[38] Radzyminski S. Legal parameters of alternative-complementary modalities in nursing practice. Nurs Clin North Am 2007;42:189–212.

[39] American Academy of Pediatrics, Section on Integrative Medicine. Mind-body therapies in children and youth. Pediatrics 2016;138(3):e20161896.

[40] Lyszczyk M, Karkhaneh M, Gladwin K, et al. Adverse events of mind-body interventions in children: a systematic review. Children 2021;8(358); https://doi.org/10.3390/children8050358.

[41] Chadi N, Weisbaum E, Vo DX, et al. Mindfulness-based interventions for adolescents: time to consider telehealth. J Altern Complement Med 2020;26(3):172–5.

[42] World Health Organization. Guidelines on the management of chronic pain in children. World Health Organization; 2020.

[43] Bohlman C. Simply be. InsightTimer. Available at: https://insighttimer.com/courtney-bohlman_wholesome-alchemy/guided-meditations/simply-be-2. Accessed August 30, 2021.

Moving?

Make sure your subscription moves with you!

To notify us of your new address, find your **Clinics Account Number** (located on your mailing label above your name), and contact customer service at:

Email: journalscustomerservice-usa@elsevier.com

800-654-2452 (subscribers in the U.S. & Canada)
314-447-8871 (subscribers outside of the U.S. & Canada)

Fax number: 314-447-8029

Elsevier Health Sciences Division
Subscription Customer Service
3251 Riverport Lane
Maryland Heights, MO 63043

*To ensure uninterrupted delivery of your subscription, please notify us at least 4 weeks in advance of move.

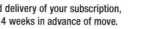